The Amino Solution

Featuring

PrescriptFit™

Products

by

Stanford A. Owen, MD

Recipes by Robert Owen

The PrescriptFit™ Medical Nutrition Therapy plan is designed for those desiring weight loss and as an aid to medical management of disease. It is not intended to replace physician management and should be used in conjunction with physician treatment and oversight. Consultation and follow-up with your physician is strongly advised prior to, and concurrent with, using the PrescriptFit™ MNT plan.

Claims of medical benefit have not been evaluated by the U.S. Food and Drug Administration (FDA). Nutritional recommendations and guidelines of the PrescriptFit™ MNT plan are compatible with most professional guidelines and recommendations.

Those with sensitivity to egg or milk products should use PrescriptFit™ products with caution as they contain egg white protein and milk solids.

Questions regarding PrescriptFit™ products or the PrescriptFit™ plan can be addressed at www.drdiet.com or by contacting us at 1-888-460-6286.

Published by:

Medical Writing and Editing:
Kathi L. Whitman, In Credible English, Kansas City, MO

Cover Design:
Eric K. Richards, EKR Creative, Salt Lake City, UT

Information Design and Desktop Publishing:
Kathi L. Whitman, In Credible English, Kansas City, MO

ISBN 978-0-9760290-0-7

Printed in the United States of America
10 9 8 7 6 5 4 3 2 1

The Amino Solution
©2009 Stanford A. Owen, MD

FOREWORD

There are a few fundamental questions that all people ask: Who am I? How did I get here? Why do I have trouble with my weight? Why do I behave the way I do? Why do I get sick? How can I get well? What happens when I die?

To a good scientist and good physician, these are questions that won't let you sleep. They keep you up at night and make your thoughts drift away during conversation.

Medical science did not evolve asking these questions. Rather, medical practice developed through trial and error. "You are sick; I treat you with this or that; you get well or not." If you get well, I try the treatment again. My great-grandfather's medical texts from the 1870s to the 1940s clearly demonstrate how our current treatment and knowledge base evolved.

Obesity treatment and nutrition therapy still use this "trial-and-error" method. Not until the discovery of Leptin, a protein (called a cytokine) made by fat cells, in the early 1990s did medical science question why a particular diet worked or failed. Why, or even if, a specific disease responded to nutrition therapy was not well studied. Routine measures of response to diet are still not routinely recorded by most physicians. Eating behavior is still considered by most to be a question of character and willpower rather than brain chemistry or metabolism.

MEDICAL NUTRITION THERAPY AND RESULTS

I started prescribing Medical Nutrition Therapy (MNT) in the early 1980s and was so drawn to the treatment results that by 1990, I decided to pursue MNT full time. I did not know why patients healed by diet change, by using nutrition supplements, or by exercising: they just did — and did so profoundly. I became compelled to know **WHY**?

The discovery of Leptin, and scores of additional cytokine proteins produced by fat cells, solved the mystery of benefits I had witnessed in my MNT patients for the past 20 years.

Today, I no longer wonder why patients improve. I no longer look at a behavioral eating problem with the prejudice of "willpower"

or character. *I understand*. Fat cells become "angry" and produce toxins when overfed, old, and misguided by diseased genes. Angry fat cells cause disease. Angry fat cells change mood and behavior. Cytokine proteins mediate that "anger."

The next 20 years of my practice will see expanded knowledge of recent discoveries. We will better understand the brain and behavior. We may further learn to improve metabolism with medication and/or nutrition. We may even crack the code of addictive behavior that plagues society from overeating to drug and alcohol abuse.

For every patient I see, the primary concerns involve whether or not a diet plan is safe, if it produces desired results, and can the patient see measurable change. For long-term change, it is important that people can register benefits to diet and behavior change each and every time they follow the plan. It is equally important the plan can be used in everyday situations and by the entire family. Above all, it must be simple, enjoyable, and reasonably affordable.

The Amino Solution achieves these goals.

THE AMINO SOLUTION AND YOU

This book offers you a usable, readable way to learn about and begin practicing the Amino Solution. Section A covers the science behind MNT and how to get ready to try this Plan. Section B offers step-by-step guidance for each food phase, including recipes, shopping lists, and cooking tips. Section C details how MNT helps reduce symptoms in a variety of common medical conditions and gives you ways to track your symptoms with your doctor throughout the Plan. The PrescriptFit™ Calendar and Amino Solution Cookbook (available at www.drdiet.com) make it easy to incorporate the Amino Solution into your lifestyle right away.

Above all, I want the Amino Solution to help you live a longer and richer life. Questions, comments? Please contact us at 888-460-6286, or visit our Web site: www.drdiet.com.

CREDITS

First, credits go to Kathi Whitman of In Credible English for an outstanding presentation of my work. If you like the style, format, ease of understanding, and ease of reading—credit Kathi. Medical professionals often have difficulty translating complicated science into understandable language and images. Kathi does this with ease and grace. In fact, I found Kathi after reading a complicated psychiatric text with perfect understanding—the first time! Thanks and congratulations to her.

My second credit goes to my son, Bob Owen, who contributed the recipes and food preparation section. Bob not only has great taste and culinary ability but a sense of commonality with the "regular guy" who wants a tasty, satisfying meal in short order. Yet, his recipes have won awards on a national television cooking show and his ability is legendary in our community. He is truly an artist in every sense of the word. His great love of life comes out in his work.

Thanks go to Anne, our clinic dietician, and Liz who were invaluable in their oversight, input, and energy. They are the guts of our program and can aid everyone interested in more information and help in reaching better health.

Also thanks to Karen and my office staff for their love and honesty toward our patients. Nothing would be possible without their tireless effort and devotion.

Finally, blessings to my wife of 35 years, Christine. Thank you for the years of understanding, honesty, vision, patience, forgiveness, and love. You are part of this manuscript at every level. Thank you. I love you.

Sincerely,

Stanford A. Owen, MD

CONTENTS

Foreword   iii

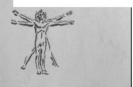

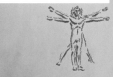

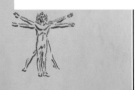

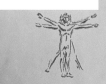

The Amino Solution
©2009 Stanford A. Owen, MD

Section C: Getting Well — Using the Amino Solution to
Treat Illness

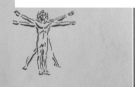

The Amino Solution
©2009 Stanford A. Owen, MD

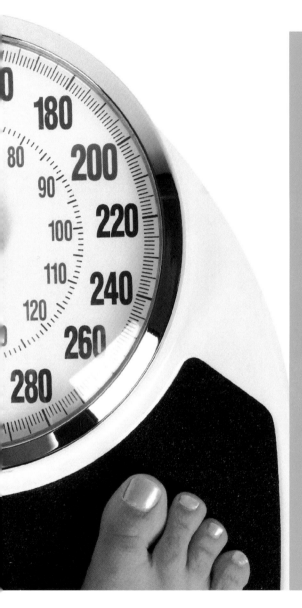

Taking Control
— Making
the Amino
Solution
Work for You

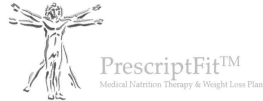

PrescriptFit™
Medical Nutrition Therapy & Weight Loss Plan

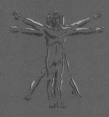

Section A: Taking Control — Making the Amino Solution Work for You

The Amino Solution, a totally different approach to losing weight and feeling healthier, relies on these key concepts:

> **The impact of amino acids (the building blocks of protein in our bodies) on wellness** — As we age and become more overweight, our bodies produce chemicals, called cytokines, at levels that cause illness. **Branched-chain and essential amino acids,** given in a precise formula, appear to improve cytokine balance and metabolism, reduce inflammation, and alleviate illness symptoms.

> **Positive reinforcement tends to change behavior** — Because the Amino Solution stresses regularly measuring results, you quickly see improvement. When you record on paper that you're taking fewer pain medications, sleeping through the night more often, or experiencing less indigestion, it's much easier to stick with what's working.

> **Real solutions need to be "real-world" solutions** — Each of us struggles with time, money, family, and work constraints that make changing eating habits difficult. The Amino Solution offers a healthy, flexible, cost-effective, and long-term solution.

> **There's more to diet success than just following a "plan"** — This approach helps you get ready for success with tips for changing your environment and habits surrounding eating as well as for talking with your doctor about the Amino Solution Plan.

Essential amino acids must be acquired from one's diet. They cannot be manufactured by the body from other proteins.

The Amino Solution's Medical Nutrition Therapy Plan stresses:

- How to reduce symptoms of illness through better nutrition

- Why flexibility in a diet plan is critical to long-term success

- How getting ready to change your eating habits is the most important "insurance" you can have for making that plan a success

- Why collaborating with your doctor and family will make seeing and feeling results more likely

The Amino Solution
©2009 Stanford A. Owen, MD

CHAPTER 1: WHAT IS THE AMINO SOLUTION?

The Amino Solution is a type of Medical Nutrition Therapy (MNT) designed to help people control a variety of chronic (and sometimes life-threatening) illnesses through diet. MNT is a process you follow to understand and control calories and caloric balancing; without such an understanding, any short-term gains you make at feeling better and/or losing weight will only be temporary.

The Amino Solution combines PrescriptFit™ nutritional supplements with MNT and a healthy dose of fun for a unique approach to feeling better than you have in years.

Although not developed strictly as a weight-loss plan, the Amino Solution uses recent medical findings about how our bodies process what we eat to solve a number of both disease- and weight-related problems.

Pages 41 through 47 offer guidance on talking with your doctor about the Amino Solution.

Two key terms you will want to remember when discussing the Amino Solution with your physician are cytokines and branched-chain amino acids.

CYTOKINES AND BRANCHED-CHAIN AMINO ACIDS — A BALANCING ACT FOR WELLNESS

In the field of nutritional science, we have learned some fascinating lessons in the last decade or two. **One of those lessons is that cytokines — proteins produced by fat tissue — orchestrate how most of our body's organs work.** These cytokines are essential to metabolism and preserve immune and organ function; however, when they become out of balance, disease in multiple organs occurs. This imbalance can contribute independently to heart disease, arthritis, depression, and injury to nerve cells and blood vessels.

The first of these cytokines discovered in the 1990s, called leptin, governs fat storage, fertility, hunger, sugar metabolism, and the immune system. Scores of cytokines discovered since leptin have equally diverse functions.

Cytokine overproduction is influenced by:

> Being overweight or obese (especially with a large belly)

> Failing to exercise regularly

Although we've known there was a link between obesity and disease for centuries, only recently have we discovered what appears to be the source of that link — cytokines.

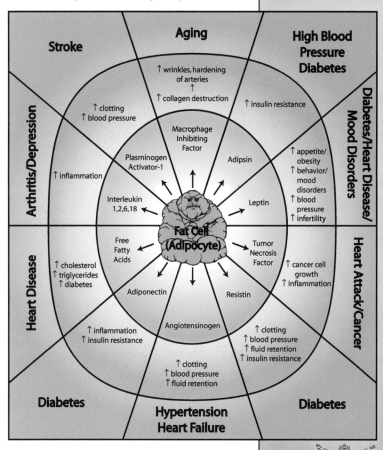

The Amino Solution
©2009 Stanford A. Owen, MD

Foods we eat without problems when we're kids may cause serious health problems in adulthood. Why? Because age and fat cell distribution accelerate cytokine overproduction, often triggering development of diseases we're at risk for based on family history.

Cytokine imbalance and its impact on feelings of hunger, satiety, cravings, and appetite may explain why some people, previously slim and trim as teenagers, only now look down at large abdomens; others may have struggled with obesity their entire lives.

> Overeating and consuming high-fat, high-calorie foods

> Aging

> Having an inherited likelihood of having certain diseases, such as diabetes or hypertension

Cytokines and Behavior — Perhaps more important than the immune, metabolic, or cardiovascular effects of cytokines are their effects on nerve cells in areas of the brain that affect our behavior. These areas of the brain control:

> Appetite

> Energy expenditure (both voluntary exercise and involuntary movement)

> Motivation

> Hunger and cravings

> Feelings of fullness

Cytokines are produced in response to your last meal as well as to your total body fat stores. They affect brain function related to feeding, explaining why one person is "stuffed" after a moderate meal while the next person returns for third servings without discomfort.

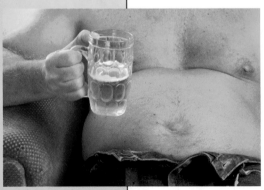

This link between behavior and cytokines explains why foods impact us differently and how we think about eating as we age. Why, for example, does a person who was previously active and vibrant, now feel sluggish and unproductive? The answer — cytokines are adversely affecting the brain AND metabolism.

Branched-chain Amino Acids (BCAAs): an Antidote for Out-of-Balance Cytokines

— The other important lesson learned from recent nutritional research is that there is a way to control cytokine imbalance through branched-chain amino acids. Amino acids are the building blocks of protein in our bodies; we don't produce those amino acids essential to this process — they must come from our diet. The term, "branched-chain amino acids," refers to the molecular structure of certain amino acids linked to reducing inflammation, improving metabolism, and fostering growth in childhood.

One of the most important findings has been that amino acids play a key role in telling our bodies how to best use insulin — a hormone secreted by the pancreas that helps the body use blood glucose (blood sugar) for energy or store it for future use in the form of glycogen in liver or muscle cells. More and more people today suffer from something referred to as "insulin resistance," which occurs when the body cells "resist" using normal or even elevated insulin secreted by the pancreas. The result is a back-up of insulin

When combined with structured food plans, specific types of protein, called branched-chain amino acids, assist in normalizing this cytokine imbalance. Branched-chain amino acids added to your diet improve appetite control and energy.

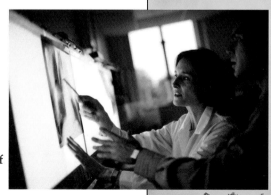

bloodstream, which is related to an imbalance in the fats stored in the blood — causing unhealthy cholesterol levels, increased triglycerides, decreased HDL (good) cholesterol. These unhealthy cholesterol levels dramatically increase a person's risk of heart disease.

While obesity and lack of regular exercise can lead to insulin resistance, important new research indicates that amino acids also play a vital role in "signaling" the insulin secreted by the pancreas to more effectively metabolize fat cells. This metabolic "signaling" is key to preventing and reducing insulin resistance and improving metabolism.

THE AMINO SOLUTION — LINKING BCAAS WITH CYTOKINES

When fat cells are "fed" balanced nutrition that contains branched-chain and essential amino acids, cytokine production improves.

Amino Acids and Medical Treatment — A number of scientific research studies have shown that amino acids play a significant role in treating many of today's most common illnesses and physical problems. Most notably, the American Journal of Cardiology published a variety of articles in 2004 that documented key research in the role of amino acids in counteracting chronic diseases, such as heart failure, type 2 diabetes and insulin resistance, and liver cirrhosis. Other research has linked depression and other affective disorders (such as schizophrenia, anxiety, ADHD, bipolar disorder, and others) in part to inflammation in the brain that may result from cytokine imbalance.

∽ Chapter 1: What is the Amino Solution? ∾

What this research tells us is that there is an apparent link between getting cytokines in balance and reducing symptoms of various physical and mental disorders.

Section B will help you easily work with structured food phases, which are key to The Amino Solution.

Using sequentially added Food Phases with amino acids helps you optimize illness treatment in new ways. For example, if you suffer from acid reflux as well as fatigue, high blood pressure and diabetes, your symptoms should all decrease significantly following the first couple of Food Phases. Then, when you add nuts (Food Phase 6), you notice that your acid reflux returns while fatigue, blood pressure, and sugar control remain perfect. When you add pork and beef (Food Phases 9 and 10), you start experiencing fatigue and your blood pressure goes up due to the effects of saturated fat, while blood sugar remains normal. Your diabetes-related blood sugar may not elevate until you add dairy products and starchy foods (Food Phases 12 and 13).

What you've learned is exactly how the foods you eat impact your symptoms AND perhaps what quantities you can have and not feel deprived. You discover that the same "damaging" food group may be well tolerated with limited exposure, so that you can regulate those damaging delights in "splurge" meals scattered throughout the month. By being sensitive to symptoms (fatigue), following signs (e.g., swelling), and checking objective measures (e.g., blood pressure or blood sugar level), patients learn to avoid harm inflicted by specific food groups.

PrescriptFit™ normalizes cytokine imbalance to control appetite, calm cravings, and diminish hunger while controlling disease.

Amino Acids and the PrescriptFit™ Medical Nutrition Therapy Plan — Modifying food intake while using the essential amino acid supplements in the PrescriptFit™ Medical Nutrition Therapy (MNT) Plan normalizes fat-cell cytokine production, improving disease symptoms and health measurements. PrescriptFit™ amino acid supplements are formulated using egg white and nonfat milk solids and are fortified with a unique formula of branched-chain and essential amino acids: leucine, isoleucine, valine, lysine, and histidine.

The PrescriptFit™ MNT Plan is a three-step approach to lifelong diet and wellness:

1. **Step One: Medical Treatment.** You will use amino acids as medical treatment for disease symptoms. Without fail, this total nutrition solution (nothing else is required besides a multivitamin) is the foundation for feeling better and losing weight.

2. **Step Two: Healing and Education.** By "phasing" in food groups, the Plan promotes healing and self education about calories and nutrition. When we focus on individual food groups for a specific time, we learn how best to prepare, eat, and combine different foods with amino acid supplements for optimum health and enjoyment.

3. **Step Three: Splurging.** PrescriptFit™ MNT makes "splurge" meals a regular part of a healthy approach to eating. NO ONE can diet forever. The Amino Solution recognizes our need to splurge; this is the diet that teaches you to manage and enjoy social eating.

Medical Treatment

The Amino Solution

Splurging

Healing & Education

Overall, the plan includes 13 Food Phases representing all major food groups. You will not be deprived of any food. Each Food Phase is built on the experience and results of each previous Food Phase. The Amino Solution allows you to design a healthy eating style to fit any taste, budget, or cultural preference.

Food Phase 1 uses food supplements containing branched-chain amino acids as total nutrition. These amino acid-containing supplements are continued with every Food Phase to normalize sugar and fat metabolism. The products also provide fullness and satiety to control appetite and cravings. By balancing cytokine production from fat cells, branched-chain amino acids influence activity of disease or behaviors deemed unrelated until now.

PrescriptFit™ Daily Dosing	
For Best Results	6-8 doses (scoops)
To Maintain Your Success	5+ doses (scoops)
Maximum Allowed (for strenuous exercise training programs)	20 doses (scoops)

Specific food categories, beginning with those with the least fat and carbohydrate count, progressing to those with the highest fat and carbohydrate content, are added to the PrescriptFit™ amino acid products sequentially. Each subsequent Food Phase teaches food science, nutrition, and culinary arts for that category.

PROVING SUCCESS — MEASURING SYMPTOM AND DISEASE RESPONSE

The Prescript Fit™ Medical Nutrition Therapy (MNT) Plan recognizes disease response to food and measures that response as a function of the diet plan. You get positive reinforcement when your symptoms improve or you gain control over your illness.

Similarly, you experience negative reinforcement when there is a relapse of signs or symptoms after adding new Food Phases, failing to take the recommended doses of amino acid product, or splurging too often. When this happens, you simply return to Food Phase I and repeat the 13-phase Plan. Even the 3-day / Food-Phase Plan will register improvement in weight and health measures.

The MNT Plan uses symptom and disease questionnaires to measure change in your health and wellness at regular intervals. This element of the Amino Solution helps to educate and motivate you for long-term health improvement. Medical conditions and symptoms improve measurably and quickly using MNT. Work with your physician to use the Symptom / Disease Questionnaires in section C to measure improvement on a regular basis. Some medical tests should be measured at physician-defined intervals. When improvements are noted, continue the Prescript Fit™ Plan indefinitely, just as you would continue to use any medication that alleviates illness symptoms.

Many different and unrelated diseases improve with MNT. It is well known that diabetes or hypertension will improve with diet intervention. Heart disease

> Most diabetics have some degree of sugar addiction. Every patient 100 pounds overweight is food addicted.

and depression may also improve with MNT since cytokines from fat tissue may contribute independently to each condition. Therefore, a particular type or amount of food may contribute to different conditions simultaneously by the same fat cell-produced cytokine. Scores of different cytokine proteins have been recently identified, each with its unique effects on different organs.

FOOD / SUGAR ADDICTION AND MNT

Addiction can be defined as the inability, despite intense mental effort, desire, and planning, to avoid a substance that causes harm. Sugar (especially refined sugar) fits the definition as an addicting substance for many, especially those with diabetes. Animal research confirms that most mammals have a preference for sweet food and, given the opportunity, will chose sugar over more "healthy" bland items every time. This research also demonstrates strong behavioral reactions to sugar-deprivation: anger, agitation, aggression, listlessness, and loss of mental acuity.

The Brain's "Appetite Center" — In the last decade, scientists have gained a better understanding of the appetite center in the brain, known as the hypothalamus. Many hormones and cytokines produced in the intestinal tract, pancreas, fat cells, liver, and muscle float via the bloodstream or send electrical signals via nerves to the brain's "appetite center." If one signal is blocked, scores of others are ready and waiting to "pick up the slack" and continue food seeking.

Taken faithfully, like a medication, these amino acid food products become a tool to aid in dietary compliance and lower food addiction feelings.

Some animals demonstrate signs of physical withdrawal and even epileptic seizures after becoming conditioned to and then quickly withdrawn from sugar.

Balancing brain chemicals that control appetite is an emerging science and art.

It is now clear that overabundance of one amino acid protein used to build brain chemicals may cause depletion of others, leading to changes in behavior and mood (such as eating to manage stress). Likewise, deficiency in the diet of a particular amino acid protein in one's diet may cause the brain to "drain" another protein to find the balance it seeks. Assuring a daily balance of these amino acids (called branched-chain amino acids) is how the nutritional food supplements in the PrescriptFit™ MNT Plan improve brain metabolism.

If MNT does not control your addiction to sugar, consult your physician about medication alternatives. Note that these medications may need to be taken throughout one's life if serious obesity exists.

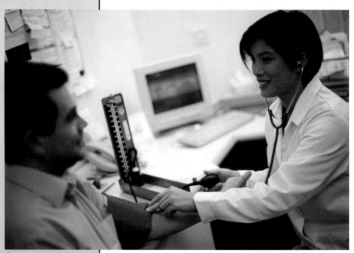

Chapter 2: Why Choose the Amino Solution?

The Amino Solution — PrescriptFit™ Medical Nutrition Therapy (MNT) — offers a world of unique advantages over other approaches to weight loss and disease/symptom reduction. It's healthy, flexible, cost effective, and designed for long-term success. Now that we know WHAT the Amino Solution involves (covered in chapter 1), let's look at WHO it's designed for as well as HOW and WHY it is successful.

1. **WHO?** — The Amino Solution is designed for those suffering from some level of obesity and specific medical conditions, which improve no matter how overweight one is or how much they lose.

   PrescriptFit™ not only improves symptoms of various illnesses, it frequently results in being able to decrease medications (only if your doctor recommends this approach), losing excess fat, and prolonging life. As you will learn in section C, medical experts recommend MNT as the first line of treatment for many medical conditions and medication add-on therapy for other conditions.

2. **HOW?** — When you are not feeling or functioning well, you want results now! The PrescriptFit™ Plan is designed to gain measurable improvement— fast! Follow the Plan precisely for best and fastest results.

Get well now, understand why later.

Unlike other diets that promote weight loss with a side benefit of feeling better, the Amino Solution focuses on feeling better with an added bonus of losing weight.

As you progress on the PrescriptFit™ Plan, note:
- What symptoms or signs improve
- How much those symptoms improve
- How fast they improve

The Amino Solution
©2009 Stanford A. Owen, MD

Patients seek physician help when they no longer feel well — when they are sick! They are happy and motivated when they improve or get well. They are less likely to want to return to that poor state of health if the improvement is substantial and measurable.

3. WHY? — Feeling well is vital for long-term motivation. Staying well requires understanding why you felt better to begin with, so you can stick with the PrescriptFit™ Plan forever. The Plan is highly educational — it gives positive reinforcement when disease or symptoms improve and negative reinforcement when symptoms return (due to abandoning the Plan or adding a new Food Phase that results in symptom return).

THE HEALTHY SOLUTION

The Amino Solution involves daily medical treatment with amino acid-based supplements. As discussed in chapter 1, these amino acids are only now being touted by the scientific community as having a "balancing" impact on the overproduction of cytokines that lead to a variety of illnesses. Using these natural amino acids rather than chemicals to balance metabolism and control hunger PLUS structured food groups that stress low-fat, low-calorie options, gives you a healthy controlled solution for today's dietary challenges.

Key components of the Amino Solution diet (using the PrescriptFit™ products and MNT Food Phases) contribute to enhanced health and wellness. The Amino Solution:

Some may want to remain in Food Phase I for several months if under close supervision by their physician.

1. **Starts with PrescriptFit™, a complete nutritional food** — One can have as much as desired and feel assured of nutritional health (a multivitamin is mandatory; physician follow up on medication and symptoms is vital).

2. **Helps fight disease using branched-chain amino acids** — Recent research links these to safely fighting inflammation, cardiac disease, metabolic disorders, and mental health problems.

3. **Doesn't eliminate any food groups** — MNT Food Phases focus on low-fat, low-calorie, structured food groups without eliminating or over-emphasizing any single food group.

4. **Lets you pinpoint were and how symptoms improve** — Measures of improvement are tracked using "clinically significant measures": lab tests your physician's office performs (e.g., blood pressure, blood sugar, cholesterol, etc.)

5. **Recommends collaboration with your doctor** — Talk with your doctor before beginning the Plan; share information from this book and discuss how to monitor symptom change as you progress through the Food Phases.

    For those with illness, physician supervision is mandatory.

6. **Is NOT exclusive** — Any and every family member can use and learn from the MNT Plan. The more you involve your family, friends, work colleagues, AND your doctor, the more likely you will be to achieve optimum health.

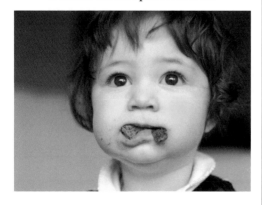

The Amino Solution
©2009 Stanford A. Owen, MD

THE FLEXIBLE SOLUTION

Forget all the "rules" of diets you've tried in the past. The Amino Solution incorporates real-world approaches that give you the flexibility to make healthy eating and wellness a permanent lifestyle change. The MNT eating Plan lets you structure:

> **How and when you consume your "treatment" doses of PrescriptFit™ supplement** — Enjoy milk shakes, soups, and puddings before meals or instead of meals every day.

> **How long you follow each of the structured Food Phases** — Introduce new food groups one at a time for three-, seven-, or fourteen-day periods designed to target the level of risk you face from illness and the rate at which you want/need to lose weight.

> **In what order you add Food Phases** — If you have allergies, are vegetarian, don't know how to cook, or just plain don't like a particular food group, you can skip or rearrange the order in which you add food groups. The important thing is to add one group at a time for the duration that fits your risk level/weight loss rate goal AND to only limit foods in Phases 9-13 to "splurge" meals (see chapter 7).

> **Eating out, at holiday gatherings, on vacation** — The Amino Solution's "splurging" concept allows eight splurge meals each month — enough to go on a cruise, spend a long weekend eating Mom's home cooking, or just maintain that Friday night pizza tradition your family adores.

> **How to improve results** — Start back at Phase 1 and try a longer duration or perhaps add more exercise or reduce the number of splurge meals per month. It's your diet, your solution.

The "splurge" concept was born of the understanding that life is unpredictable. "Stuff" happens. Schedules go by the wayside. Partying occurs. Tragedy hits. Events occur in our lives every day that are more important than the next meal or recipe preparation. The ultimate flexibility — "falling off the wagon" — is NO BIG DEAL with the Amino Solution. When people have too many splurge meals or don't stick to the initial phases of the Plan, it's NO BIG DEAL. You just get back on the program and move on. The Amino Solution is a learning experience, not a "pass" or "fail" test. In fact, your body will tell you what to do. For most people, symptoms such as pain, inflammation, acid reflux and others quickly return when they either fail to maintain amino acid supplement intake and/or indulge in too many high-calorie/high-fat meals. Relief comes quickly once you get back on the Plan.

This is the only diet that not only recognizes that we all have to splurge from time to time, the Amino Solution gives you a simple way to manage and ENJOY those times.

There are times in our lives when our kids, our parents, our jobs, our friends all have a major impact on when, how, what, and where we eat.

REAL-WORLD FLEXIBILITY

1. **Don't avoid eating out.** Once you've completed the first two or three Food Phases (based on how you choose to structure them), you will be able to go out to any restaurant and enjoy poultry, seafood, vegetables, salads, nuts, fruit, and eggs in any quantity you wish.

2. **Having a busy week with lots of overtime at the office?** PrescriptFit™ shakes, puddings, soups, and snack bars are an easy, "no-brainer" way to stay full, satisfied, and feeling great. Then, when the deadlines are over, enjoy that "splurge" meal you've not had time for. The Amino Solution is the flexible solution designed for your unique lifestyle.

The Amino Solution
©2009 Stanford A. Owen, MD

Pick the Phase Duration that's Right for YOU			
Level of Risk/ Weight Loss Rate (estimated pounds/ week depending on initial wt.)	**Medical Health**	**Days/ Phase**	**Medical Attention Needed During MNT**
Low/Slow (1-2)	• Not taking prescription medication for specific illness • Conditions not yet life-threatening	3	
Medium/ Moderate (2-3)	• Taking prescription medications for chronic illness • Have significant symptoms • Stable and not at risk for imminent death	7	• Need frequent monitoring of condition • Should be managed by a physician during MNT
High/Rapid (3-6)	• Taking prescription medications for chronic illness • Have symptoms that are disabling and require frequent physician exams • At risk for death or serious disability	14	• Need frequent monitoring of condition • MUST be managed by a physician during MNT

THE COST-EFFECTIVE SOLUTION

All weight-loss diets cost money for special foods/supplements, "membership," and/or coaching. The Amino Solution involves a cost for purchasing the PrescriptFit™ supplement products; however, using these products is less expensive overall than following other commercial diet plans we've compared. Realize that some diets structure costs based on complete foods provided, others include fees for participation in the program, and others allow for purchasing your own food (at grocers or in restaurants) for some or all meals. The table on page 26 presents some of the monthly costs involved with the Amino Solution as compared to Weight Watchers®, NutriSystem®, Jenny Craig®, Atkins®, or South Beach® diets; outside food purchases will vary.

What do we actually spend on the food we eat? Both the U.S. Department of Agriculture and the Food Marketing Institute estimate that the average family spends between $500 and $1,000 per month with food prepared at home, not including eating out. The Restaurant Association estimates that half of all meals are eaten out of the home in most urban settings, which might raise the family expenditure to about $1,300/month.

> *Eating costs us money, no matter how you look at it.*

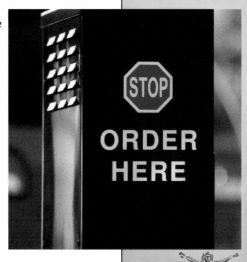

If you use PrescriptFit™ shakes, soups, or puddings to replace one or two meals each day ($2-4/meal), you will save considerably over "normal" diets and fast food ($4-8/meal).

Given these figures, PrescriptFit™ products are significantly less expensive than the average North American food bill (groceries plus dining out). Fast food or restaurant food is considerably more expensive.

But, won't adding all those "healthy" fresh foods to the PrescriptFit™ meals cost a lot more at the grocery store? You are right that many foods — seafood, fresh fruits and vegetables, whole grains, and low-fat dairy items — typically cost more than high-fat, high-calorie processed foods. In fact, according to a study published in March of 2005 by the University of California Agricultural Issues Center, the higher cost of healthier food choices is equal to about $32-$41 a week for consumers. Some of the cost involved food items just not being available in easily accessible stores; some cost reflected simply higher prices for the healthier item due to volume of product sold. What's the solution if you're on a limited budget? Consider your current spending each day for food and try this experiment:

1. Replace one meal a day totally with a PrescriptFit™ shake, pudding, or soup.

2. Have a PrescriptFit™ shake, pudding, or soup right before you eat a regular meal, which will reduce the amount you want to eat during that meal.

3. Control portion sizes and stop eating when you are no longer hungry.

If you track what you actually spend with this approach, you may very well find that healthier eating isn't more expensive after all.

But what about your overall budget? How much do you currently spend on medications — both prescription and over the counter?

How much do you spend out of pocket each year on medical office visits related to chronic illness? It is very likely that, because balancing cytokines with amino acid supplements reduces symptoms of many chronic illnesses, you will start to see some significant savings in medical costs. No doubt about it — chronic illness is an expensive way to live!

What would feeling better mean for your productivity at work and at home? What could that productivity mean in terms of career advancement? Although we may not be able to put a dollar figure to these considerations, we all know that when we feel good, everything just goes better.

THE LONG-TERM SOLUTION

The Amino Solution offers a unique approach to weight loss and wellness that helps people make permanent lifestyle change vital for living longer, more productive lives.

How? The PrescriptFit™ MNT Plan:

> *Avoids deprivation* — No foods are excluded permanently.

> *Lets you eat the size portions you want* — If you use the PrescriptFit™ supplement shakes, puddings, and soups as medical treatment **before and/or instead o**f some meals, you can eat all you want of the foods allowed in whatever Phase you are currently in.

> *Gives you something "to look forward to"* — MNT let's you consistently add Food Phases, teaches you how to prepare foods in new ways that taste great, and allows eight "splurge" meals a month after completing Phase 8.

The Amino Solution is one of the best investments you can make in your health and your future. It pays back astonishing dividends!

The Amino Solution
©2009 Stanford A. Owen, MD

> *Keeps you from getting bored* — MNT holds your interest by focusing on measures, providing new methods of food preparation, and improving taste and variety.

Well-known weight-loss diets share a number of attributes, but studies of successful outcomes point to certain factors that appear to ensure long-term success. These factors are:

> Exercise

> Fruit and Vegetable Intake

> Group Attendance

> Supplement (Shake) or Special Food Product Compliance

> Record Keeping

Of these, supplement (shake) compliance was the stronger predictor of success, statistically, than all of the other four factors combined. Given these "success factors," compare the Amino Solution with other well-known diet approaches (see the table on the next page).

The Amino Solution's unique nutrition treatment strategy is:

> Safe
> Medically credible
> Satisfying
> Easy
> Socially acceptable
> Instructive
> Intuitive
> Inexpensive
> Reproducible
> Measurable

Comparisons of Popular Commercial Diets				
Diet	Portion Control	Group Support	Carb Control	Packaged Meals
Atkins			✓	
Sugarbuster			✓	
Weight Watchers	✓	✓		✓
South Beach			✓	✓
Zone	✓		✓	
Jenny Craig	✓	✓		✓
HMR/Optifast	✓	✓		✓
Amino Solution			✓	✓

	Shakes[1]	Diet Behavior Tracked[2]	Symptom Outcomes Tracked[3]	
Atkins				
Sugarbuster				
Weight Watchers		✓		
South Beach				
Zone				
Jenny Craig				
HMR/Optifast	✓	✓		
Amino Solution	✓	✓	✓	

1. *In outcomes data collected, supplement (shake) compliance was a stronger predictor of success, statistically, than all of the other 4 factors combined.*
2. *In outcomes data collected, the five variables predicting long-term diet success in order of greatest impact on success) are: supplement (shake) compliance, exercise, record keeping, group attendance, and fruit/vegetable intake.*
3. *Only Amino Solution tracks clinical endpoints for disease symptoms. Amino Solution allows individual patient tracking for 21 medical conditions as well as psychological, quality of life, and eating behaviors (national Web-based data available at www. drdiet.com).*

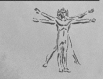

The Amino Solution
©2009 Stanford A. Owen, MD

COST COMPARISON FOR COMMERCIAL DIETS

WEIGHT LOSS PROGRAM	BASIS OF COST*	ESTIMATED MONTHLY COST**
The Amino Solution	Meal Replacement PrescriptFit™ Product ($2–4/meal)	If meal replacement PrescriptFit™ used as complete nutrition, ~$240/mo
Weight Watchers®	Own food Meeting fee ($11/week); online consultation (~$19/month)	$63/month (includes no food costs)
NutriSystem® (NS)	Purchase NS Foods plus own vegetables, fruits, milk NS Foods (28-day program) $289–337/month	$289–337/month
Jenny Craig® (JC)	Purchase JC products ($11–19/day) Meeting/consultation fee ($6/week)	$336–576/month
Atkins®	Own food or meal replacement shakes, bars (~$2/meal)	$180/month (figures for comparison ONLY; meal replacement products NOT recommended as sole diet)
South Beach®	Online program ($5.00/week) Own food or convenience foods made by Kraft (average cost $5.00/meal)	$470/month (based on online program plus 3 Kraft meals/ day)

* Basis of costs are published information at the time of publication
** Monthly costs are IN ADDITION TO groceries purchased and/or restaurant dining on one's own, if applicable to the program. Where program offers meal replacement products, those have been figured at the programs specified monthly cost or at 3 meals/day for 30 days for comparison. Specific diet programs may prohibit making meal replacement products the sole diet; consult your physician before structuring any diet plan.

Chapter 3: How to Ensure Success

Adequate preparation for permanently changing your diet, nutrition, and overall health is a big step. It requires several adjustments — in your attitude and perceptions, in your environment, in your day-to-day routines — that are critical to your long-term success. For many, dieting becomes a roller coaster of short-term change and long-term failure because they just weren't ready to make the changes the diet they chose required.

Getting Your Head in the Game

How we view what we eat or choose not to eat has a great deal to do with our attitudes and perceptions about food. First of all, remember that the word, "diet," is not about how much you eat; it is about what foods you eat. What each person eats, when they eat, where they eat, and how they view these factors are very personal considerations. Improving our diet is all about balancing who we are, how we feel, and how we look with our eating habits.

It's important to realize that your general eating patterns and habits are greatly influenced by your upbringing. What time of day you choose to eat lunch or dinner, whether or not you eat snacks, whether or not you eat quietly or in big, family meals — all these factors are influenced by what you've grown up with. If mom's or grandma's special meals featured fried meats, lots of starches, and a bounty of yummy desserts, you probably keep those traditions sacred with your own families. Kids growing up in

The experiences you've had to date with "dieting" have been different than those you will experience with the Amino Solution.

The combination of amino acid supplements, structured food groups, and "legal" splurging gives you unprecedented ability to feel full and satisfied while eating less, not have to control portions in any Phase, be flexible in ways that fit your lifestyle and tastes, and never feel deprived.

These differences spell a whole new experience with diet.

> *Eating patterns, likes and dislikes, and family routines develop early and are very difficult to change.*

households where parents don't particularly like or prepare vegetables, fish, whole grains, and fruits will likely not fix those foods themselves when they become adults. There are also numerous emotional ties between love and food — approval for cleaning our plates, food as rewards for good behavior, comforting routines that include bedtime snacks.

Add to these challenges, the fact that our bodies change as we age, metabolizing the same foods differently. Also, the food industry has undergone tremendous changes, making a wealth of processed foods more available and less expensive over the past 50 years. All these packaged foods are heavily marketed and easily accessible to us every day. With our busy schedules, it's less likely that people will prepare and eat home-cooked fresh foods on a regular basis.

Its no wonder so many people feel that they've failed to change their diets.

Failure to control your weight is NOT a failure to avoid pleasure (greed) or to be disciplined (control of instinctual behavior), and it does not mean that you lack intelligence. Failure to control weight is a complex issue that involves environmental, emotional, hormonal, instinctual, and motivational factors that cause more calories to enter your body than are being expended. Period.

The solution: Accept that failure is normal and must be confronted. Accept the challenges you've taken on and allow for the realities of your environment. Take the self-quiz on pages 30–31 to determine your specific challenges and how you might overcome them.

The Amino Solution
©2009 Stanford A. Owen, MD

EXERCISE 1: DIET-CHANGING CHALLENGES AND STRATEGIES

Pinpoint Your Specific Challenges	Strategies for Success
LIKES AND DISLIKES	
• List foods you don't think you can live without: _____ _____ _____ • List 3 types of foods you don't care for: _____ _____ _____	• Use splurge meals to enjoy must-have foods. • Learn to prepare one new food a week in a different way that might taste better. Use your Amino Solution recipes and advice on shopping and seasoning each Food Group to "train" your palette.
CLEAN-PLATE OBSESSION	
Do you always feel like you need to finish everything on your plate? _____ (yes or no)	• Use smaller plates. • Prepare/serve smaller servings. • Dish plates in the kitchen and immediately put excess food away instead of using serving dishes that make having "seconds" possible. • In restaurants, have the server bring a "box" for half your meal BEFORE you start eating.
FOOD FOR REWARD	

Do you save desserts, treats for rewarding yourself when finishing a project or accomplishing something difficult?
 	
_____
(yes or no)
	• Determine three, non-food rewards (e.g., hot bubble bath, going to the movies, calling your best friend long distance) to substitute for food. List these below:
	  1. _____
	  2. _____
	  3. _____
	
	• Use food rewards as splurge meals, reserving your very favorite treat eaten in a special place to make the reward even better.

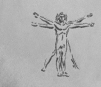

Section A: Taking Control...

EXERCISE 1: DIET-CHANGING CHALLENGES AND STRATEGIES, CONT.

SOCIAL EATING

Do your social commitments include frequent dinner parties, family food events, or eating out? _____ (yes or no)	• Always have a PrescriptFit™ shake or pudding with at least 2 scoops of supplement powder BEFORE each social eating event. • If your plate comes prepared, divide the foods in half and only eat that portion. Ask to take the other half home as leftovers (throw away the leftover box at home before putting it into the refrigerator). • If there is a buffet, use a salad plate instead of a dinner plate. If tempted to go back for more, go outside for a walk or leave the party early. • Try to join groups/activities that don't include meals. • Count each social meal as a splurge meal (8 per month allowed) and only attend the amount of events allowed. • Look for a friend or family member that also attends these functions to be your coach and ally. This will also help you be more accountable for your food choices at these events.

SNACKING

How often do you snack? __Not every day __About once a day __Between meals all the time __At bedtime What are you doing/feeling when you eat snacks? __Watching TV __Working at a desk __Feeling bored __Socializing with friends __Other?_____	• Plan another diversion that keeps your hands busy (e.g., play solitaire, knit, go for a walk) for the times you know you're likely to snack. • Don't ever buy or store high calorie/high fat snacks. Keep fruit, nuts, and cut up veggies on hand for snacking. • Try suggesting that socializing with friends be done during a walk or other activity that doesn't involve food. • Take regular, short breaks from work to avoid boredom and the desire to snack. • Substitute 8 ounces of water or a PrescriptFit™ shake or pudding for a snack.

The Amino Solution
©2009 Stanford A. Owen, MD

Now let's focus on our goals; envisioning why we're doing battle with these lifestyle changes will help keep a positive perspective on the process. With the Amino Solution, you develop new discipline because you acquire new knowledge and skills, you have built-in accountability, AND you practice these new habits over time without fear of failure.

Whether throwing a party or just planning for daily snacking, replacing sugar snacks with fruit will cause less resistance from kids and spouses.

EXERCISE 2: IDENTIFYING YOUR GOALS

WHY AM I DIETING

To look better:
__Be more attractive to a partner
__Be more accepted by family
__Be more accepted by friends
__Be more accepted at work
__Other?

To feel better:
__To help treat current medical problems
__To feel more energetic
__To reduce back/joint pain
__To enhance sports performance/increase stamina
__Other?

WHAT ARE MY PRIMARY GOALS?

Weight: _____
Shape (inches of waist, hips, etc.): _____
_____
Posture: _____
Clothing sizes: _____
Prolonged life (to what age): _____
Financial viability (% of increased productivity): _____
Reduced medical costs (in $$$ or % of annual expenses): _____
Reduced disease symptoms: _____
Quality of life (physical, social, emotional): _____

ADDING KNOWLEDGE SEQUENTIALLY ABOUT FOOD GROUPS, PREPARATION, TASTE

Myths and misinformation about foods abound. These focus on (high fat, low fat), food supplements or additives, artificial flavorings, or salt and sweeteners. Many people get sidetracked by these myths and avoid making changes in their diet or revert to familiar eating patterns out of fear or misinformation. In the exercise below, test your current knowledge about food myths.

See pages 53 through 54 for answers to Exercise 3: Myth or Fact?.

EXERCISE 3: MYTH OR FACT?	MYTH	FACT
1. There are "good" and "bad" calories.	❏	❏
2. If a food has more saturated than unsaturated fat, it means that there are more calories per ounce in that food.	❏	❏
3. I can eat more and not gain weight if I load up on protein.	❏	❏
4. You have to quit eating starch and fat to ever lose weight.	❏	❏
5. Vegetable oil is better for you than oils made from animal fat (e.g., lard).	❏	❏
6. Salt is bad for you; it should be avoided in any diet.	❏	❏
7. Artificial sweeteners are safe to use.	❏	❏
8. Sugar-containing beverages are the number one cause of obesity in Western culture.	❏	❏
9. Even moderate alcohol intake will cause weight gain.	❏	❏
10. Condiments should always be avoided to ensure diet success.	❏	❏
11. There's no way you can lose weight without reducing portion size.	❏	❏
12. You can eat two times as much seafood and poultry than beef and pork without gaining weight.	❏	❏

The Amino Solution
©2009 Stanford A. Owen, MD

Some people simply refuse to learn new tastes, experiment with new flavors, methods of food preparation, or new buying habits because they just don't want to change. Change, by definition, is stressful.

Medical nutrition, obesity, and food science researchers are in closer agreement about the kind of nutrition therapy used in the Amino Solution. There is an explosion of new information in every scientific journal. Some of this information is delivered by "sound bites" on the television or delivered out-of-context in newspapers, magazines, and via the Internet. We all "inhale" this scant new information as gospel, remember bits and pieces, and fixing these bits as fact into our memories.

Each Food Phase of the Amino Solution MNT Plan addresses that category of food with the latest science, nutrition, and calorie math. Each Phase provides best culinary methods for that food choice.

The result — accurate decision-making when choosing food for yourself or family while quickly preparing more scrumptious meals.

Try not to get sidetracked by food and diet myths; you're eating based on the latest discoveries in nutrition science.

Results = Knowledge X Skill X Accountability X Practice Over Time

The Amino Solution
©2009 Stanford A. Owen, MD

Practice the skills you learned in previous Food Phases until you master them. Each time you use a recipe from a previous Food Phase, re-read that Food Phase.

**Learn.
Reinforce.
Practice.
Teach!**

Managing food for health just takes practice!

LEARNING ABOUT NUTRITION, FOOD BEHAVIOR, PREPARATION, AND "ACCOUNTING"

Skills are learned. Most people learn eating habits, cooking skills, and nutrition "science" from parents or friends. Nutrition information in school is presented haphazardly and is often obsolete or single-minded. Nutrition classes rarely teach culinary or cooking skills. Each Food Phase of the Amino Solution MNT Plan teaches skills you need for purchasing, preparing, and consuming foods that promote wellness.

BUILT-IN ACCOUNTABILITY ENSURES THE BEST RESULTS

We all perform better when we're held accountable for our actions. The Amino Solution provides built-in accountability to help you succeed with weight loss and symptom reduction.

Accountability factors include:

> **Recording your progress on your PrescriptFit™ calendar** — Do it religiously. Don't lie or fudge. Learn from your efforts.

> **Relying on meal replacement use** — The more PrescriptFit™ shakes, soups, or puddings you use, the more you will lose and the better disease improvement you will experience. Studies show meal replacement use is the #1 predictor of diet success in our modern world.

> **Getting regular exercise** — Daily Over Duration! Do some exercise every day. Daily exercise of short duration will produce superior weight loss and

medical benefit than the same total exercise done two or three times per week.

> **Involving others** — Connect with your physician, sponsor (who you buy PrescriptFit™ products from), or friend/coach. Have an important person review and accept your written results (on the calendar and questionnaires) and review your progress with you.

Learning the MNT Plan

When you start on the Amino Solution, you will probably want to order:

- The PrescriptFit™ Calendar — An invaluable tool for long-term success with the Amino Solution

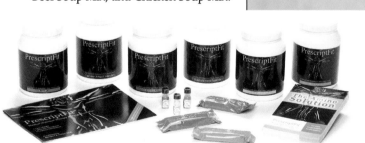

- A three- to four-week supply (depending on use) of PrescriptFit™ products — the Vanilla Shake/Pudding Mix (regular or lactose-free formula), Chocolate Shake/Pudding Mix (regular or lactose-free formula), Beef Soup Mix, and Chicken Soup Mix.

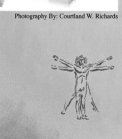

Photography By: Courtland W. Richards

- An assortment of delicious, calorie-free flavorings

The Amino Solution
©2009 Stanford A. Owen, MD

THE PRESCRIPTFIT™ CALENDAR

The Calendar provides space for you to record key factors related to the Plan each day, including:

- What Phase of the diet you are currently in

  - The number of doses (scoops) of amino acids you consumed in PrescriptFit™ shakes/puddings/soups

    - Time you spent exercising

      - If you used a splurge meal (> Phases 9-13)

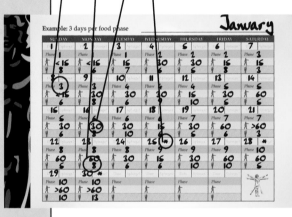

Keeping consistent, accurate records of how you progress on the Plan will help you pinpoint what causes improvements or relapses you experience.

Other pages of the Calendar provide:

- A place to record baseline information

- Symptom Score Sheets to record your results every four weeks or after each phase

PRESCRIPTFIT™ PRODUCTS

The PrescriptFit™ products are nutritionally complete supplements that come in vanilla or chocolate (lactose-free formulas available) for shakes and puddings as well as both a chicken and a beef soup mix. All mix with water (and crushed ice in the case of shakes) and are exceptionally flavorful without additional enhancement. All PrescriptFit™ products are formulated using egg whites and nonfat milk solids, and are fortified with additional branched-chain and essential amino acids: leucine, isoleucine, valine, lysine, and histidine. ("Essential" means the body cannot manufacture these amino acids from other dietary proteins).

When using the Vanilla shake/pudding mix, take your favorite glass, fill 1/2 with water and 1/2 with ice; pour into blender with 2 scoops of Vanilla. Blend until creamy. Add another scoop for an "ice cream" like effect. This product is delicious as creamer for coffee, when mixed with diet soft drinks, as a topping

Those who see the best results from the Amino Solution are those that consume more than six doses of PrescriptFit™ supplement each day.

Blender Tip:

Most blenders sold for non-commercial use are not designed for multiple use per day, especially when blending liquids with ice.

To avoid burning out the motor of your home blender, be sure to use only crushed ice and to never use more ice than water in shake preparation. Should you experience problems with blenders, consider purchasing a commercial bar blender (designed for daily, high-intensity use) from a restaurant supply company.

For a less expensive alternative, appliance repair persons recommend finding a blender that is at least 25 years old at a garage sale or used appliance store.

Apparently, they don't make 'em as good as they used to.

for your favorite fruit, or with nuts (Phase 5). The Chocolate shake / pudding mix is made from the finest imported cocoa and can be mixed the same as the Vanilla for optimum texture and flavor.

The Lactose free varieties of Vanilla and especially the Chocolate are very rich tasting. Use the Chocolate alone for maximal "chocoholic" satisfaction or mix with one scoop of Vanilla for a milky chocolate delight. Lactose free is the preferred product for those with irritable bowel syndrome (IBS).

The soup mixes include the same nutritionally complete formulas and are also fortified with branched-chain essential amino acids. The Chicken Soup is great as a hot drink or can be used as a thick sauce for meat or vegetable dishes. Beef soup gives a full-bodied beef taste that is especially good with meals or as a hot drink. Mix a scoop of each together for a real treat. Add vegetables, seafood, or poultry to the soup mix when you get to those Phases.

Other products included in the PrescriptFit™ line include specialty soup mixes and a variety of snack bars. Visit www.drdiet.com for more information.

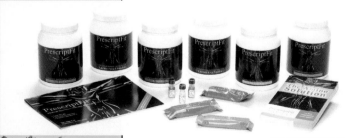

Photography By: Courtland W. Richards

The Amino Solution
©2009 Stanford A. Owen, MD

FLAVORINGS

PrescriptFit™ flavorings are sugar-free, fat-free ways to bring fun variety to your shakes and puddings. Highly concentrated, these flavors encompass almost any taste — fruit, citrus, caramels and butter pecan, amaretto and Bavarian cream, mint chocolate, English toffee, chocolate hazelnut — you name it. Use these flavorings to experiment with new toppings for fruits, blender drinks (if adding alcohol, don't try this until Phase 11), and varied milk shakes and puddings. Visit www.drdiet.com for more information.

ENVIRONMENTAL "CLEANUP"

For a few weeks before you begin the Amino Solution Plan, it's a good idea to do what we call the "Environmental Cleanup." This involves five crucial steps:

1. **Replace tempting foods not part of Phases 1-8 with the foods allowed during these Phases.** Success is more likely if tempting foods are not in the immediate environment — your home, workplace, and automobile. Alcoholics and cocaine addicts know relapse to drug use is more likely if they frequent situations where alcohol or cocaine is present. Food today tastes better than ever, is inexpensive, and is everywhere. No wonder many patients tell me they are food addicted and feel like they have no place to hide.

2. **Continue your usual diet pattern for four weeks BUT add in three doses of PrescriptFit™ shakes, soups, or pudding mix in a single serving BEFORE (or instead of) breakfast and three doses in a single shake, soup or**

Be sure to remove ALL sugared drinks from your environment, including soda, juice, milk, and sports drinks. They are truly "empty" calories. Diet soda, sugar-free ice tea, and coffee with artificial sweetener and fat-free, non-dairy creamer are allowed during any Phase of the Amino Solution.

Those who see the best results from the Amino Solution are those that get more than 15 minutes of exercise each day.

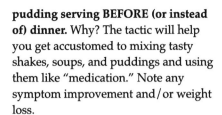

pudding serving BEFORE (or instead of) dinner. Why? The tactic will help you get accustomed to mixing tasty shakes, soups, and puddings and using them like "medication." Note any symptom improvement and/or weight loss.

3. **Do not change your exercise habits** (or lack thereof), but be sure and note what those habits are each day along with your weight. When you make a change in your exercise habits, you will want to compare results with this baseline condition.

4. **Measure your pre-Plan symptoms on the first Symptom Score Sheet located in the back of the Calendar.** You will use the second Symptom Score Sheet (and copies of it) to record symptoms and evaluate change after four weeks on the Amino Solution Plan (and at four-week intervals thereafter).

5. **Collaborate with your doctor to ensure that your experience with the Amino Solution is healthy** and successful (see the next section). Get your doctor's advise on which Plan (14-day, 7-day, or 3-day per Phase) to choose for the health and weight loss goals you determined in Exercise 2 on page 31.

For a comparison of each Plan, see page 20.

TALKING TO YOUR DOCTOR ABOUT MNT

Most physicians receive very limited training on treating disease with diet. Medical schools don't emphasize nutrition or medical nutrition therapy as part of their regular curriculum. Once in practice, physicians learn from popular diet books or from professional publications, which contain bits and pieces of nutrition-related material.

When asked for diet advice, most physicians refer to local dieticians or recommend a popular book. Some refer to commercial diet programs such as Weight Watchers. Ask. Share your Calendar and this book with your physician and ask his/her opinion. Show him/her the Physician FAQs on pages 44 through 47 and the journal articles in appendix C. Have them contact us with questions at 888-460-6286.

Be sure to:

1. **Make an appointment with your doctor** BEFORE beginning the Amino Solution Plan. Take this book and your Calendar, discuss the Plan, and review your current state of health including any baseline measures (blood pressure, weight, waist measurement, fasting blood sugar, cholesterol, triglycerides, etc.) that you will want to track as you proceed with the Plan. Use Exercise 4: Talking with Your Doctor on the next page to plan for covering important items during this initial visit. Many of the questions reflect current health guidelines. Write down your doctor's answers to each question.

2. **Use the Symptom/Disease Questionnaire** score sheets (in your Calendar and section C of this book) that you and your doctor agree best reflect the measures you should follow. Most score sheets require you to reevaluate symptoms after Phase 1 and after every four weeks. Refer to the individual score sheets for more detail.

Medical professional organizations recommend diet treatment of disease as the initial primary treatment for a number of medical conditions. Conditions or symptoms listed in the Amino Solution materials reflect these professional guidelines as well as extensive publication, outcomes data, and/or experience.

The important thing is to embark on the Amino Solution WITH your doctor. You are not just trying to lose weight; you are actively pursuing health and reducing or eliminating symptoms of chronic illness. How your body reacts and what impacts that reaction might have on prescription medications you're taking demands close collaboration with your doctor.

If you choose the high-risk (rapid weight loss) approach, talk with your doctor about more frequent contact.

3. **Make a follow-up appointment** four weeks past the time you begin the Amino Solution. Review the results you've recorded on your Symptom/Disease Questionnaire score sheets with your doctor to evaluate what impact the changes you've made are having on your symptoms.

4. **DO NOT discontinue or alter the way you take any prescription medications,** even if your symptoms disappear. Always contact your doctor before making any changes to medications.

EXERCISE 4: TALKING WITH YOUR DOCTOR

Instructions: Check off those questions you want to ask your doctor at your next appointment. Take along a note pad to record his/her answers.

❑ What is your experience with medical nutrition therapy?

❑ What diet recommendations do you currently make? To whom do you refer patients for nutritional counseling?

❑ What impacts might MNT have on me personally given my health and current medications?

❑ What baseline measures on the Disease/Symptom Questionnaires can be monitored over time for improvement?

❑ Are there other measures I should monitor?

❑ What is my body mass index (BMI) and is this a problem for me?

❑ What is my waist circumference and does it possibly signal insulin resistance problems?

❑ Are my triglycerides over 150 mg/dL?

❑ Is my HDL cholesterol less than 40 (men) or 50 (women) mg/dL?

❑ Is my blood pressure greater than 130/85 mm Hg?

❑ Is my fasting glucose greater than 110 mg/dL?

❑ Should MNT be a first-line treatment for my problems? Or, add-on treatment?

The Amino Solution
©2009 Stanford A. Owen, MD

PHYSICIAN FAQs

How fast does one see responses?

Responses vary depending on the medical condition and its severity, additional illnesses, and medications prescribed. The more severe the symptoms, the faster and more dramatic the response. Those individuals with few medical problems and a minimal amount of weight to lose will note the least dramatic "benefit." Most symptoms respond within several weeks.

Which diseases respond most predictably?

Using over a decade of practice-based experience and measuring outcomes data, we've found diseases that usually respond quickly and dramatically are Type 2 diabetes, GERD (acid reflux), edema (swelling), fatigue, dyspnea (breathlessness), CHF (congestive heart failure), and irritable bowel syndrome. Slower and less-dramatic responses occur with steatosis (fatty liver), headache, joint and back pain, hypertension, hyperlipidemia, and sleep apnea. Least-predictable improvement occurs with asthma, angina, arthritis (inflammatory type), depression, fibromyalgia, and insomnia.

What are expected side effects of the diet, and how are they managed?

Most common side effects are gas and diarrhea, managed by using Lactose Free PrescriptFit™ products. Weakness occurs when blood pressure or diabetes medications are not tapered or stopped fast enough. Most physicians are surprised by the degree and rate of improvement and often cite "the diet" rather than the necessary medication adjustments when side effects occur. Constipation is occasionally a problem, usually solved by adding fiber (Citrucil), stool softeners, or Fish Oil (Omega III). Laxatives are usually unnecessary. **(See Appendix D for more information.)**

How does this diet compare to traditional national dietary guidelines? How does it differ and are those differences a problem?

The Amino Solution reflects traditional nutrition guidelines by promoting leaner foods for everyday consumption. The differences are sequentially adding food groups and lack of portion control. The sequential strategy can be safely used since the PrescriptFit™ products provide complete nutrition. Portion control is unnecessary since the PrescriptFit™ products taken prior to meals result in less total calorie consumption and improved metabolism of foods consumed. Another important difference is that the diet fosters learning about food group nutrition while experiencing how adding each food group impacts medical symptoms.

The Amino Solution
©2009 Stanford A. Owen, MD

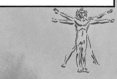

Physician FAQs, CONT.

When is close physician supervision recommended/required?

Whenever a medical condition exists that requires adjustment of medication, especially diabetes, congestive heart failure, hypertension, and edema (swelling). These conditions require close monitoring and medication adjustment. Other medical conditions usually need adjustment less urgently. **Monitor all individuals following the 14-day/Phase Plan.**

How can a physician contact us with questions?

Anytime. Via www.drdiet.com or by phone (888-460-6286), contact with physician or dietician professionals is always available. A direct call will always be answered or returned.

What published findings support this approach?

A number of journal articles have been published on specific impacts of amino acids and cytokine imbalance on specific diseases (e.g., metabolic syndrome, type 2 diabetes, cardiovascular disease, mental health disorders). These articles have been included in the Bibliography at the back of the book (see "Resources for Your Doctor" area on pages 243–251). Unfortunately, most of this research has not focused on disease versus specific diet approaches, and no diets have been researched with multiple diseases concurrently. Few have correlated specific changes in cytokines with specific diseases using a specific diet. Published research does not seem to reflect what Dr. Owen has done in the past decade — look at multiple diseases, measure specific cytokines (mostly CRP), and do so on a diet time line (most measure weight loss as the measure of benefit rather than symptom reduction).

The Amino Solution and the PrescriptFit™ products were developed by a physician in private practice who is also a physician nutrition specialist (see "What is a Physician Nutrition Specialist" FAQ on the next page) without funding from major pharmaceutical companies or food manufacturers. The cost of performing scientific studies that would satisfy publication requirements for most peer-reviewed journals is astronomical. However, efforts are underway to secure grants for formal studies since the impact on health is, in our opinion, so substantial for such minimal cost and risk.

Physician FAQs, CONT.

What practice-based findings promote the Amino Solution?

In 1995, Dr. Owen started measuring multiple end points when patients followed the HMR very low calorie diet (VLCD). By 1997, he had a large enough experience base (>1,500 patients) to start a computer-based data system. By 2000, he had measures on all the disease parameters covered in section C of this book. As data emerged demonstrating benefit of branched-chain amino acids, the PrescriptFit™ products were developed to maximize and improve outcomes seen with the VLCD plans. Data since 2000 has been collected using the progressive PrescriptFit™ Food Phase plan with similar results.

How were the Clinical Outcome Measures developed?

In the early 1990s, Dr. Owen's clinic developed a computerized data entry system to measure improvement in disease conditions witnessed daily. The data allowed a more objective way to prove the benefit and to improve methods and products. After development of measures for the obvious disease targets, they realized that many less-obvious conditions and symptoms responded as well. The result of the data system is the Symptom Score Sheet used in the PrescriptFit™ Calendar.

What is a Physician Nutrition Specialist?

A Physician Nutrition Specialist is someone who has studied in the field of nutrition for a specified time, has contributed to the nutrition sciences on a professional level, has passed a Board Certification Exam, and then been accepted by that Board as a Certified Member. Dr. Stanford Owen was one of fewer than 100 physicians certified in the initial board applications of 2001, the first year of formal Board formation. He is accepted as a Fellow in the North American Association for the Study of Obesity — an honor requiring that one contribute significantly to the published, clinical, or socioeconomic issues relating to obesity and nutrition. Few Board Certified Physician Nutrition Specialists have developed commercially available nutrition therapy plans. None have measured outcome as a component of a medical nutrition therapy program — Dr. Owen's life-long mission.

What medication-balancing issues are important for patients using MNT?

For patients taking medication for diabetes, hypertension, or fluid retention, the need to down-regulate these medications occurs rapidly, and patients will get symptomatic (even dangerously symptomatic) if not monitored closely.

PHYSICIAN FAQs, CONT.

What role do the individual food phases play in diet success and symptom mediation?

Sequentially adding each food group promotes education: learning how each food group specifically impacts medical symptoms and how to buy, cook, and flavor specific foods for a specific time period. This education promotes long-term eating habit changes and validates the patient's experience about what makes them feel better and what doesn't.

Additionally, each food group has nutritional characteristics that predict benefit or harm to physiology (in terms of calories, percent protein, percent fat and type of fat, percent carbs and type of carbs) — all specific to individual physiology. For example, a patient who is diabetic with hypertension and high lipids might hate vegetables and seafood. His wife wants to be a vegetarian. This could pose a real dilemma for adding some of the food groups; however, the built-in flexibility of the Amino Solution allows for skipping some of the early Food Phases or reordering them to accommodate these types of dilemmas.

How often should follow-up appointments be scheduled for patients on MNT?

Follow-up appointments should be scheduled weekly for more serious medical problems requiring medication adjustment as well as for those that choose the 14-day/Phase Plan. Follow-up on a less frequent basis will be adequate for less compelling problems and those choosing the 7-day or 3-day/Phase Plans.

What branched-chain amino acids are used in PrescriptFit™ products?

Although the ratio is a trade secret, all of the branched-chain and essential amino acids are used in the PrescriptFit™ products.

OVERCOMING OBSTACLES

Know the obstacles to improved health from the "get-go." The greatest obstacle to most is the food environment provided by loved ones: spouses, children, parents, and friends. We are literally "loved" to death with food in modern culture. Parents would never think of offering their drug-addicted teen more addictive drug, yet those same parents allow their socially shunned, obese child to consume foods likely to cause obesity.

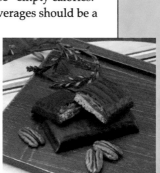

Willpower just doesn't work.

In my experience, most patients feel their own medical problems are not the concerns of others. "It's my problem, not yours," and "You should not have to suffer for me," are typical "martyr" statements. Likewise, many patient family members feel exactly the same —"It's your problem, not mine." In reality, everyone pays for chronic disease and misery related to obesity via the monthly health insurance bill as well as physical, mental, or social disability.

The Amino Solution allows every major category of food. The only food group that you should completely avoid is sugared beverages (soft drinks, juices, sport drinks, and milk). There are NO redeeming features to anyone consuming these "empty calories." Avoiding these caloric beverages should be a family affair.

Family members are often more reluctant to remove bread, snacks, crackers, cakes, pies, and pasta compared to caloric beverages from the household. Alternatives (fruit, vegetables, and PrescriptFit™ snack bars) should be discussed and negotiation must occur. You will need to communicate to family members that "willpower" cannot overcome tempting delights. It is relatively easy to say "no" to bringing a pie into the house. It is impossible not to eat the pie once in the house.

PLANNING FOOD / PRODUCT PREPARATION

In section B, you will find that each Food Phase discussed includes tips for shopping, buying, seasoning, and preparing foods within that Phase. Review these and use the "shopping lists" provided for Phases 1-8 recipes to get started creating the pantry items you need to make the Plan a success.

Revisit the organization of your kitchen. Perhaps you have a cabinet or other space you can devote completely to your PrescriptFit™ product prep. Gather together your blender, measuring cups/spoons, PrescriptFit™ shake and soup mixes, flavorings, and condiments (such as fat-free, sugar-free Jell-O and pudding and other seasonings) in a single location to make it easy to quickly prepare your PrescriptFit™ doses. No one wants to take the time to pull out and replace all these components if scattered about the kitchen.

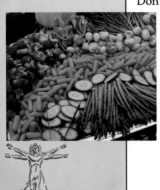

Don't let yourself run out of essentials. There are too many high-fat, high-sugar alternatives just around the corner that take less time to pick up than going to the grocery store. Be sure to stock up each week on what you need for the Food Phases your currently working with.

PLANNING FOR EXERCISE

Exercise recommended for the PrescriptFit™ MNT Plan is very simple. After years of treating patients, both successfully and unsuccessfully, I've learned that exercise is a major predictor of weight loss success. As you would expect, those who do the most exercise most consistently lose the most weight, improve the most medically, and decrease the most their need to take medications.

What might seem somewhat paradoxical is that the amount of exercise is not as important as the consistency of exercise. Those who do any amount exercise every day will generally have better outcomes than those who exercise a few times per week, even if that exercise is considerably more intense and more prolonged.

Modest walking produces health benefits nearly as great as with intense exercise. The key words are "health benefits." Having a "buffed" and lean body may take large amounts of daily exercise, but health improvement can be registered with much less effort.

Be sure to record your time spent exercising each day on your PrescriptFit™ Calendar.

The Amino Solution
©2009 Stanford A. Owen, MD

Muscle manufactures and alters cytokine production. Daily muscle use affects daily cytokine metabolism.

The Amino Solution suggests doing 15 minutes of exercise per day, preferably broken into two or three separate sessions of five to 10 minutes each for greatest benefit.

Why would such meager activity bring health results?

1. **"Daily" is a key theme in exercise.** Daily performance of any health habit shapes the day with compliance of other health habits, like compliance with diet.

2. **Five to 10 minutes will never interrupt other activities**; thus, the excuse that "I just don't have time" tends to go away.

3. **Fifteen minutes is equivalent to walking one mile.** One mile is a measurable number and is the "payback" number (100 calories burned) we use to emphasize calorie value in food. Is one glass of juice or a bowl of cereal once per day worth 1.5 miles (150 calories) of walking payback per day? I doubt it!

4. **Fifteen minutes adds up to total fat loss.** One mile of walking per day (15 minutes) burns 100 calories in a 150-pound person. That adds up to 2800 calories per month. One pound of fat contains 3500 calories. Therefore, the 150-pound person would burn up about 8 pounds per year (and the 300-pound person 16 pounds per year) with 15 minutes of exercise per day. In five years, 40 pounds would be lost.

Learning to use exercise time most productively is important. Exercise devices can be helpful for those in hot, cold, or rainy environments. They are inexpensive. **Buy them and use them daily!**

If the fifteen minutes are used to improve postural strength, such as abdominal strengthening exercises, you will realize additional benefit for painful and damaged back and joint structures.

The Amino Solution
©2009 Stanford A. Owen, MD

WORKING WITHIN YOUR LIFESTYLE

Okay, so you might wonder how to make the Amino Solution work for you if you travel extensively for business, work in a location where food preparation isn't really possible, or just don't know anything about cooking.

The built-in flexibility of the Amino Solution is designed for success no matter what life throws at you. In any case, you will probably need to start Phase I of the Plan when you can be at home for the first couple of days at least. This will let you prepare the shakes/puddings as often as necessary using a blender and crushed ice and adding allowable flavors from your pantry. Of course, this will be more of a challenge if you select the 7-day or 14-day Plans; however, once you go off to work, the Soup mixes can be mixed in a cup with water and heated in the microwave for lunch. You can make a shake or two ahead and freeze, letting it thaw to the right consistency by mid morning.

By following the cooking instructions in each of the Food Phases in Section B, you can know very little about cooking and learn just a few skills to make following the Amino Solution Plan a success.

One of the best ways to overcome dislike of cooking is to take one day a week and find a friend to cook with. Make larger quantities of soups, fruit salads, and baked/grilled dishes that you can "warm up" after work during the week. Enjoy the time together and learn from one another. You can also do this with your own family, creating some new quality time that promotes mutual understanding about foods and healthy eating patterns.

If you tend to eat out fairly often, use some of the strategies in the "Tips for Business Travelers" (below) to make dining out work for you.

The Amino Solution offers a great deal of flexibility for any lifestyle challenges you currently face. You can choose the number of days per Phase, the order in which you add Phases 2-8, and when to plan your "splurge" meals.

TIPS FOR THE BUSINESS TRAVELER

- Create a small bag with individual servings of PrescriptFit™ product and small flavoring bottles to take with you on the road.

- Consider purchasing a MagicBullet® blender (sold in various retail stores and over the Internet at www.buythebullet.com). It is small, lightweight, and very powerful.

- Once you've hit Phase 2 and beyond, scope out restaurants in the areas you travel (online or from feedback from business colleagues in that location) that cater to those on low-fat, low-calorie diets. For example, some restaurant chains feature entrees with specific calorie, fat, and WeightWatchers® point totals. Call ahead and ask about grilled fish or chicken entrees as well as steamed vegetable plates; when you arrive, be sure to request your meals without sauces but with lemon wedges or salsa or Tabasco sauce.

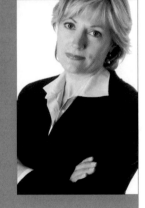

- Almost every town has a grocery store with a salad bar; try getting a salad WITHOUT cheese and high-calorie/high-fat dressing to go and picnicking in a nearby park.

- If your travel budget allows, ask to stay in "suites" hotels that feature in-room microwaves and refrigerators; stock up on fruit, shrimp cocktail, or microwavable grilled chicken wings to have in the room (depending on the Phase you're in).

The Amino Solution
©2009 Stanford A. Owen, MD

ANSWERS TO EXERCISE 3 (PAGE 33): MYTH OR FACT?

1. MYTH — Calories are "worth it" or "not worth it". Calories have no "character" — they are not "good" or "bad." A calorie is a unit of heat liberated from food during digestion used for energy, growth, and repair. There are only two things you need to remember about food calories:
   - Proteins and carbohydrates contain 4 calories/gram.
   - Fat contains 9 calories/gram.

2. MYTH — There are few differences in types of sugars, proteins, or fats relative to calories. All fat, saturated or unsaturated, solid or liquid, hidden or obvious, contains 9 calories per gram.

3. FACT — When you eat protein in excess, it is converted either to carbohydrate for energy or to fat for storage. The "conversion" of protein to carbs or fat "uses up" 25 percent of calories in the protein molecule. Therefore, one can "cheat" on protein calories by 25 percent and not gain weight. Remember, that's just one-quarter more in your serving — not double the portions you usually have. In addition, protein does not stimulate the abnormal release of insulin and fat cell-produced cytokines, and therefore may not aggravate diabetes, pre-diabetes, hypertension, and lipids (cholesterol).

4. MYTH — While it is vital to minimize over-use of carbohydrates and fats that are most likely to cause abnormal metabolism and obesity, sumptuous foods must be a part of quality life. That is the Amino Solution difference. By planned splurging on 8 of 90 meal slots per month, little long-term damage will happen to weight loss or health goals, but a lot will happen to long-term diet compliance and happiness.

5. FACT — Unsaturated fat made from vegetable oil is less "toxic" to the cardiovascular system than saturated animal fat. Animal fat harms arteries and metabolism. Still, even unsaturated fats need to be consumed in moderation.

6. MYTH — Salt is not harmful except in specific medical conditions, such as congestive heart failure (see section C). In fact, cytokines are much more likely than salt to cause fluid retention, which is why adding amino acids can be so effective in reducing fluid retention. Salt has no calories. Salt tastes great, especially when combined with other herbs and ingredients, making "new" foods taste more like what you're used to.

7. FACT — Scientific research does NOT support the claims that artificial sweeteners can cause harm. In fact, the harmful effects of sugar far exceed those reported at times with saccharin or aspartame. Saccharin no longer contains health warnings since science has demonstrated no risk for long-term consumption. Aspartame (Equal®) has not been found to cause harm either. Articles suggesting aspartame causes formaldehyde accumulation are not supported by science.

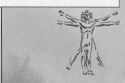

Alternatives include Splenda® or stevia. Splenda® is a product developed from natural sugar containing no calories; however, it may not be appropriate for diabetics. Splenda® mixes well with beverages and doesn't break down when heated on the stove, in the oven, or in the microwave. Stevia, a plant-based substance, has been used for centuries to satisfy sweetness cravings and is growing in popularity as an artificial sweetener.

8. FACT — Soft drinks, juice, sport drinks, and milk should be eliminated permanently for those suffering from obesity and related illness. Juice often contains more sugar calories than soft drinks. Nonfat milk or skim milk contains very little fat and is a healthy food product; however, those with serious obesity often over consume milk, so it is best eliminated.

9. MYTH — Alcohol in moderation (as part of a splurge meal) does not pose a significant problem unless you suffer from diabetes or cardiovascular illness. Alcoholic beverages are allowed in the Plan once you reach Food Phase 11 (to allow your metabolism to become more balanced). If you can't avoid regular alcohol intake until Food Phase 11, you should talk with your doctor about the potential impacts of regular alcohol consumption on your overall health.

10. MYTH — Although many popular condiments should be avoided because they are high in fat (cheese, cream sauces, gravy, salad dressings) or contain high concentrations of sugar (catsup, cocktail sauce, barbecue sauce), many condiments can produce health benefits. Mustard, catsup, vinegar(s), Creole mustard, horseradish, even nuts are all allowed as condiments with the Amino Solution. Because condiments enhance taste, it is important to use them wisely to get more enjoyment from the healthy foods your body needs. Thankfully, most popular condiments now offer nonfat or no-sugar alternatives and new products appear frequently. PrescriptFit™ recipes help you learn to use herbs, vegetables, artificial sweeteners, and plant "stanol" butter for flavoring.

11. MYTH — Although portion size contributes greatly to obesity, requiring specific portion sizes and /or weights for each meal makes following a diet very difficult for many people. MNT controls calorie intake by using amino acid products to satisfy hunger while allowing low-calorie foods in large portions. If you have a PrescriptFit™ shake before dinner, you will not be as hungry and will likely take smaller portions without having to "measure" or feel guilty. Add to that the ability to eat an unlimited amount of the foods in the Food Phases you've completed. "Splurge" meals without portion limits are used for high calorie, high fat, high sugar foods rather than limiting portions. Eight splurge meals are allowed per month from Phases 9-13.

12. FACT — Seafood and poultry have ¼ to ½ the calories of beef and pork. Using seafood and poultry as primary meats for most meals limits calories. One pound of seafood contains 400 calories. One pound of beef or pork contains 2,000 calories.

NOTES

NOTES

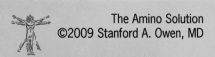

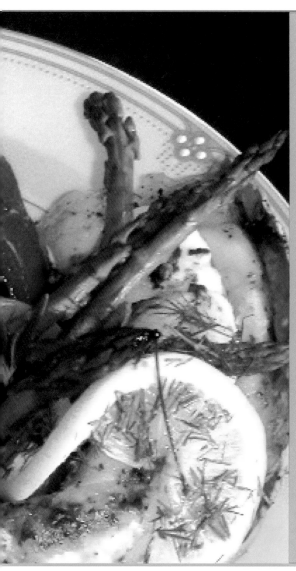

*Diving In —
The Structured
Food Phase
Approach*

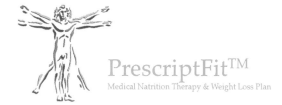

PrescriptFit™
Medical Nutrition Therapy & Weight Loss Plan

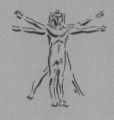

Section B: Diving In — The Structured Food Phase Approach

Chapter 4: Overview of the Food Phase Strategy

Think of the Amino Solution Food Phase strategy as a personal training regimen, in which you work with YOU – your own personal trainer – one step at a time, building new skills and experience, until you have achieved your desired level of fitness. What could be easier and more personal than having yourself and your own body as your trainers!

You will start at the beginning with the first food phase and gradually add food groups in each subsequent phase until your food plan includes all major food groups. You will not be deprived of any food. Each time you transition to a new food group, your body will communicate with you, the trainer, about its experience. Your body will tell you which foods make you feel more or less energetic, which relieve or exacerbate symptoms, and which cause you to lose or add weight. Just as a personal trainer adjusts exercise strategies for an athlete, you will be able to adjust your food plan for optimum health.

The Amino Solution puts you in charge. You can design your own eating styles to fit any taste, budget, or cultural preferences. The sample recipes in this chapter will help you envision the possibilities and may be used as a guide to get started.

The Amino Solution's Medical Nutrition Therapy stresses:

- A Food Phase strategy that allows you to isolate those foods that most impact how you feel

- PrescriptFit™ supplements that both taste great and dramatically reduce a number of illness symptoms

- A healing and education period that lets you learn to adjust your buying, seasoning, and cooking habits for optimum health

- An oh-so-needed splurge element that gives you opportunities every week to eat socially and to treat yourself to the things you love

The Amino Solution
©2009 Stanford A. Owen, MD

⮞ Section B: Diving In... ⮜

Throughout this section, you will find brief stories of people with different lifestyles who have found their own ways to successfully adapt the Plan to their particular realities of work, home, family life, and travel.

In Phase 8, you will add PrescriptFit™ snacks, which will replace old, empty-calorie habits with nutritious snacks.

Think of Food Phase 1 as the all-important conditioning phase for your new eating regimen. You will use PrescriptFit™ food supplements containing branched-chain and essential amino acids as total nutrition. These supplements – in the form of tasty shakes or soups – are continued with every Food Phase to normalize sugar and fat metabolism. The products also provide fullness, satiety, and control of appetite and cravings.

Phases 2–8 will be your education and healing phases. One at a time, you will add the most important nutritional food groups – seafood, poultry, vegetables, eggs, nuts, and fruit – beginning with food groups containing the least fat and carbohydrate, progressing to higher fat and higher carbohydrate. In each new Phase, you will learn food science, nutrition, and culinary arts for that category. In Phases 1–8, you will find yourself healing – eliminating the toxic cytokines you've built up from eating poorly.

Finally, in Phases 9–13, you will gradually add the higher fat and higher calorie components of a complete lifestyle diet. By this time, you will be ready for an occasional splurge day (see chapter 7). By being sensitive to symptoms (fatigue), following signs (swelling), and checking objective measures (blood pressure or blood sugar level), you will learn to avoid harm inflicted by specific food groups. That's why it's very important to experience each Phase in a prescribed sequence.

Medical Treatment

The Amino Solution

Splurging

Healing & Education

Each Food Phase is designed to teach you a fundamental principle: How your body reacts to different food groups. By following the plan and eating only the foods listed in each Phase, you'll learn what your body needs.

"But I hate seafood," you're thinking. Or, "I love dairy products." If you want to gain control of your health, you need an open mind about the variety of foods available. On the other hand, if you have food allergies, or if you have chosen a vegetarian lifestyle, this book will suggest ways to modify your eating plan to accommodate those needs.

Variety in food groups and methods of preparation will help you feel more satisfied and be more successful. For example, if you think grilled catfish can be the only item you will eat during Phase 2 (seafood), you're not realistically accounting for the variety that is surely part of your current life. Realistically, you will quickly tire of grilled catfish and will be tempted to find variety in something other than what is outlined in the Phase. If this is you, you're missing your opportunity to gain control of your health, and you may be setting yourself up for failure.

As you begin each Phase, you'll be reminded of the diet components that you will use consistently throughout the Plan and beyond as you maintain your weight. And, you'll be reminded to use your PrescriptFit™ Calendar to record your splurge meals each week.

Are you ready to get started? If so, let's take a tour of the 13 PrescriptFit™ Food Phases, starting with Food Phase 1 geared especially for medical treatment.

To ensure variety in your personal experience, each Phase includes these tools and helpful hints for increasing your food options without compromising taste or your success:

1. **The grocery list** — What to buy to get you started with the sample recipes included in this section, as well as staples (such as seasonings) that will help you create recipes that fit you and your family's needs. The grocery list will be included in Phases 1–8, when you are, perhaps, learning to experiment with new foods and recipes. In Phases 9–13, you may choose to experiment with new recipes or return to some "family favorites" for your splurge meals. Therefore, we have not created a grocery list for these Phases.

2. **Taste tips** — Brief notes on seasonings, spices, and how to use them to vary some of the basic recipes.

3. **Sample recipes** — Basic recipes for each phase.

Chapter 5: Medical Treatment with Amino Acids — Food Phase 1

No one likes to be told they're getting old or out of shape, but our metabolism will tell us the truth whether we like it or not! Obesity, age, and/or genetic predisposition often contribute to metabolic disorders. And many diseases related to diet have common genetic patterns. Recently, scientists have discovered new pieces of the metabolic puzzle related to fat cells, which:

- Produce abnormal proteins called cytokines that disturb metabolism

- Release cytokines into the bloodstream in response to the size and content of meals

- "Talk" constantly to the brain and other organs via the bloodstream and nerve fibers

The good news is that you can regulate the type of cytokine production by the amount of specific nutrition you feed your fat cells. That's exactly what Medical Nutrition Therapy (MNT) enables you to do. People who are sickest gain the most dramatic benefit. Even those expressing mild fatigue and "tiredness" are shocked at how much better they feel and how fast they improve.

Medical Treatment

The Amino Solution

Splurging

Healing & Education

WHY YOUR OLD DIET DIDN'T WORK FOR LONG

High protein, low-carb, and very low calorie diets (VLCD) diminish cytokine production; however, long-term compliance with these diets is difficult. Consider, for example, the popular Atkins diet. Unlimited amounts of protein and fat help dieters feel full and satisfied while allowing brisk weight loss. And, to the surprise of nutrition scientists, Atkins dieters experience improvement in some medical conditions. However, nutritionists question how much long-term artery damage may result from the high-fat, high-protein combination. Studies have shown that less than 10 percent of Atkins dieters have continued the program for more than a year.

VLCD dieters also experience metabolic improvement using shakes only. The most difficult variable to predict in any individual dieter is: At what caloric level and with what foods does metabolism again slip back toward disease? Dieters following VLCD plans precisely (prior to PrescriptFit™) experienced different rates of relapse. Some simply binged out, bailed out, and bombed out, resulting in total and immediate relapse of

Phase 1: PrescriptFit™ Shakes, Puddings, Soups

their symptoms and disease. Others "re-fed" perfectly according to the plan. Even with the "perfect" dieters, it's impossible to accurately predict when or if they will relapse and what condition will relapse first.

While many thousands of successful VLCD dieters are still off most medications and vitally active years after serious, chronic diet-related illness, thousands is not good enough. Every person can experience long-term diet success and good health. Until development of the PrescriptFit™ MNT Plan, no simple, logical, nutritionally and socially acceptable diet plan existed that could work with every patient and every family.

THE PRESCRIPTFIT™ ADVANTAGE

The PrescriptFit™ MNT Plan offers you multiple advantages over traditional diets:

- Amino acid supplements that regulate metabolism and banish cravings

- An easy-to-follow food plan that you can customize to your lifestyle

- Education and tools for long-term maintenance

- Measurable health improvements

You'll see results right from the start. Food Phase 1 of the PrescriptFit™ MNT Plan focuses on the amino acid supplements that provide complete nutrition as well as a satisfying taste and a feeling of fullness. Only the supplements are used for nutrition in Food Phase 1 (plus a daily multivitamin); no other food is allowed.

Depending on the rate at which you want to lose weight and/or improve symptoms, you can choose to stay on Food Phase 1 for three,

PrescriptFit™ is a food-based amino acid supplement that tastes great, is filling, and is inexpensive —especially when compared to today's pharmaceutical and hospital costs.

seven, or fourteen days. The longer you stay on this phase, the faster you may expect to see improvement.

If you are taking medications, you must ask your health care provider to monitor changes in your condition.

If you choose shorter Food Phase intervals yet do not achieve your weight or medical goals, simply repeat the 13 Food Phases at the same or longer intervals until you achieve your goals.

PrescriptFit™ products are formulated using egg whites, nonfat milk solids and fortified with additional branched-chain and essential amino acids: leucine, isoleucine, valine, lysine, and histidine. ("Essential" means the body cannot manufacture these amino acids from other dietary proteins). Use of five or more doses guarantees a perfect balance of each amino acid per day. We recommend six doses as the minimum daily amount. Eight doses is optimal, but no overdose is possible. Twenty doses is the maximum recommended, even for those in strenuous exercise training programs. Do not take less than 6–8 doses per day during Food Phase 1 unless you are under a medical practitioner's care and supervision.

PrescriptFit™ normalizes cytokine imbalance to control appetite, calm cravings, and diminish hunger while controlling disease.

PRESCRIPTFIT™ DAILY DOSING	
For Best Results	6–8 doses (scoops)
To Maintain Your Success	5+ doses (scoops)
Maximum Allowed (for strenuous exercise training programs)	20 doses (scoops)

The Amino Solution
©2009 Stanford A. Owen, MD

Section B: Diving In... ◦

You'll find the exclusive use of PrescriptFit™ amino acid products in Food Phase 1 not only results in weight loss, symptom relief, and medical improvement, it also avoids confounding or confusing excuses for failure, such as Aunt Sue's pie or a bag of chips.

Rather than sabotaging your success with extraneous foods, use Food Phase 1 to concentrate on how much and what medical measures (e.g., blood pressure, cholesterol, weight) and symptom measures (e.g., reduced pain, better sleep, more energy) begin to improve.

Some people ask, "What if I want to just stay with Phase 1 for an extended period of time?" If you have a more serious illness, you may continue use of amino acid supplements, without additional food, to normalize metabolic abnormalities as you adjust medication. Just be sure to continue to take a daily multivitamin and stay in close contact with your physician. If you use PrescriptFit™ products exclusively for more than four weeks, please ask your doctor to monitor your condition weekly.

PrescriptFit™ products come in a variety of flavors, all of which contain similar doses of branched-chain amino acids. You can alternate flavors through the day or week, or stick to one flavor, most commonly chocolate or vanilla, using different flavorings (listed on the next page) to provide variety during the week.

In Food Phase 7, add fresh, canned, or frozen fruit to your shakes for a real treat. Avoid canned or frozen fruit preserved with sugar.

Supplement your PrescriptFit™ products with at least five, eight-ounce glasses of water or calorie-free beverages each day.

You may even mix diet soft drinks with the PrescriptFit™ product (try Diet Coke® or diet root beer with the vanilla PrescriptFit™ to make a "float").

Be sure to take a daily multi-vitamin while using the PrescriptFit™ plan. If you were already taking vitamins or dietary supplements, you may continue to take them if your health practitioner agrees.

Amino Acids as Treatment — Measuring Results

PrescriptFit™ products improve metabolism. You'll be able to measure results by symptom, physical, or laboratory improvement. As with any medication that provides benefit, PrescriptFit™ products can and should be used forever at five or more doses per day. If you discontinue the amino acids and resume the eating habits that originally caused the illness, symptoms will relapse.

If necessary, you can begin Food Phase 1 over again (and again, and again) if symptoms or diseases relapse and weight gain recurs. Relapse may occur with a particular food that you add during one of the Food Phases. Or, you may relapse months, even years later, if you revert to old eating habits. If this happens to you, simply go back to Food Phase 1 and start over, adding new Food Phases after control of your symptoms or conditions. If you responded the first time, you should respond again. With time and experience, you'll recognize the food category culprit(s) contributing to relapse, and you'll learn to avoid them.

PrescriptFit™
Amino Acid Varieties
- Vanilla Shake
- Chocolate Shake
- Lactose Free Vanilla Shake/Pudding
- Lactose Free Chocolate Shake/Pudding
- Chicken and Beef Soups

THE GROCERY LIST

This is not intended to be an exhaustive list of possible products you can add to PrescriptFit™ products. Use your imagination – if it doesn't contain fat or sugar, you can add it!

ADDITIVES FLAVORINGS PUDDING MIXES

- Jell-O™-Brands (Sugar-free only)
- Watkins™ specialty flavorings and herbs
- Spices (cinnamon, pumpkin pie, nutmeg)
- McCormick® flavorings
- Crystal Light" soft drinks
- Tea or coffee — Mix sugar substitute, PrescriptFit™ vanilla flavor, and a bit of water for coffee creamer

TASTE TIPS: ADDING FLAVOR, VARIETY, COLOR, AND TEXTURE TO PRESCRIPTFIT™ PRODUCTS

You'll want to experiment with adding a variety of sugar-free flavorings to your PrescriptFit™ products. Remember, variety will prevent boredom and encourage your continued success with the Food Phase plan. If you experience demonstrable health improvements using PrescriptFit™ products, you'll want to continue them forever, but not if you're bored. Your "Grocery List" (at left) lists possible additives.

To obtain optimal flavor:

- Fill the glass or cup with ice and/or water first then fill with water, no matter the size of the glass. Add 1–3 scoops of PrescriptFit™ (1 for a small cup, 3 for a large glass/cup). Blend for two minutes for a creamy shake, one minute for an icy shake.

- PrescriptFit™ amino acid shakes will stay blended (hot or cold) in a thermos.

- PrescriptFit™ amino acids are stable when frozen or heated. For great treats and desserts (especially for kids, teens) use wooden sticks and plastic popsicle molds for frozen treats. Try chocolate and Crystal Light flavorings.

- For a thicker shake, add additional powder, more ice, and blend for a longer time. Egg whites cause the product to "soufflé" into a creamy delight with prolonged blending.

- Hot drinks (hot chocolate and soups) are best blended first in hot water. Prolonged microwave heating may result in coagulation of the egg whites.

~ *Chapter 5: Medical Treatment with Amino Acids* ~

Loretta — A Family Success Story

When Loretta came to the clinic, she was a 40-year-old mother of three teenage boys and had gained 35 pounds with each pregnancy and an additional 20 pounds since the youngest was born 13 years ago. At 280 pounds, she now suffered from diabetes, hypertension, severe back and knee pain, and was constantly exhausted due to sleep apnea. Out of "love" for her children, Loretta has denied no foods or snacks to the entire family. Consequently, all but one child (and her husband) are substantially overweight.

Loretta was referred by her physician, who gave her less than five years to live if she didn't get her health and diet under control. After a lengthy discussion about the difficulty and commitment necessary to lose 130 pounds and some problem solving with the dietician, it was decided she would prepare meals from Phase 1–8 for her children while using the 14-day per Phase plan (a total of 26 weeks to complete all 13 Phases). Her boys could use shakes and snacks as desired. The family reluctantly agreed to remove all snacks and calorie-laden drinks from the house, including milk and juice (two "sleeper" obesity-causing beverages). The PrescriptFit™ shakes have ample calcium, even for growing boys. She bought an ample supply of snack bars and shakes to prevent anyone in the family from feeling deprived.

Loretta practiced recipes from each of the first eight Phases for most meals and prepared two "splurge" meals per week for the entire family, usually mid-week and on Sunday. This prepared Loretta conceptually and practically for each Phase. On Saturday, her kids went out with friends for pizza or burgers.

Her husband bought her a stationary bicycle with arm attachments, a used treadmill, and exercise ball for less than $500, which she used every morning. He agreed to walk with her every afternoon for 15 minutes or longer. She rarely recorded less than 30 minutes of exercise per day on her PrescriptFit™ Calendar.

Loretta achieved complete remission of her diabetes within two weeks (never to return), discontinued blood pressure medication by four weeks, resolved her back and knee pain by 12 weeks, and lost a total of 140 pounds. Her family collectively lost 70 pounds (husband lost 40 and the kids lost about 10 pounds each).

The total cost of the weight loss Phases was less than the medication cost and doctor visits of only the prior six months (just her insurance deductible, not the actual cost). With good planning, open communication, and love, Loretta and her family were successful.

Case Study

The Amino Solution
©2009 Stanford A. Owen, MD

Optimal results occur when PrescriptFit™ shakes or soups are used prior to or with a meal in future Food Phases.

Experiment with timing.

- Keep your PrescriptFit™ product next to the blender at home or work.
- Take one or several large thermos containers to work or in the car.

PHASE 1 RECIPES

SHAKES — DOSING AND MIXING

Vanilla or Chocolate (regular or lactose free)

1. Fill a 12oz glass with ice and water and pour into a blender.

2. Add 2-3 scoops of PrescriptFit™ and blend. Continue to add powder and/or ice to reach desirable thickness, taste, and texture. Some like crunchy ice shakes. Others prefer smooth and thick shakes like those from fast food restaurants. The most important point is to experiment with how you like your product to taste. Remember to use 6–8 doses (scoops) per day in Food Phases 1–13.

3. To make more flavorful shakes, simply add your favorite spice or flavoring toward the end of blending.

PUDDINGS — DOSING AND MIXING

Lactose Free Chocolate and Vanilla make perfect puddings in 30 seconds!

1. Place 1–3 doses (scoops) in a cup or bowl.

2. Drizzle in water while stirring until the desired texture of pudding is reached.

3. For variety, add spices, nuts (Food Phase 5), or nonfat whipped cream (Food Phase 12). Puddings are great for treats on-the-go and quick clean up.

SOUPS — DOSING AND MIXING

The chicken and beef soups are spicy, but you can mix them to suit your taste.

1. Start with 1 cup of hot water and mix (with a whisk) or blend.

2. Add ½ scoop when first mixing and an additional ½ scoop until desirable taste is achieved. Mixing one scoop of Beef Soup with one scoop of Chicken Soup produces a delightful blend.

Soup Additives/Tips:

- Bouillon cubes, granules, or liquid varieties, such as beef, chicken, fish, shrimp, ham, or vegetable

- Salsa — except calorie-adding varieties that contain oil, sugar, or beans

- Dehydrated vegetables — onions, mushrooms, etc.

- Dry seasonings (any variety) — try basil, thyme, oregano, garlic, etc.

- Fresh, frozen, or canned vegetables, seafood, chicken, pork, or beef at appropriate Phases for body, texture, and flavor

Now you're ready for the Education and Healing Phases of the Amino Solution.

Cooking Tip:
Once you reach the later Phases, pour the PrescriptFit™ soup over vegetables or meat dishes as a gravy. Or, you can mix soups very thick and spread lightly over vegetable dish as a casserole.

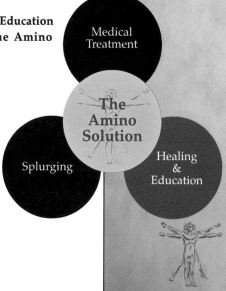

Chapter 6: Healing and Education — Phases 2–8

Phase 2 Seafood

Seafood is one of nature's most perfect foods, especially for those with chronic medical conditions related to diet. Seafood is virtually 100 percent protein and contains minimal fat, with the exception of certain fish (tuna, salmon, sardines, mullet, mackerel) that contain Omega 3 fatty acids, which are beneficial to the cardiovascular system and brain. Due to the low-calorie content of seafood, it is virtually impossible to "overdose" on seafood and gain weight unless large amounts of butter or oil are mixed with the fish.

> **Dosing:**
> There is no restriction on amount or type of seafood allowable per day on the PrescriptFit™ MNT plan. Neither health or weight gain concerns are an issue. All you can eat! Enjoy!·

Seafood Choices — Fish (fresh or saltwater), Shrimp, Crab, Lobster, Crawfish, Oysters, Mussels, Clams

Seafood is satiating because protein does not stimulate hunger-causing insulin, takes longer to digest, and tastes great. Seafood does not stimulate toxic cytokines.

However, seafood does not contain essential vitamins found in vegetables or fruit; therefore, vitamin supplementation is essential

Phase 2: Seafood

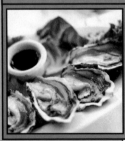
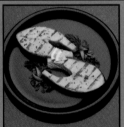
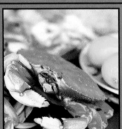

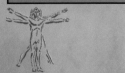

if a "seafood only" diet is utilized with PrescriptFit™ amino acids.

Seafood Myths

Cholesterol — Shellfish contain cholesterol-like molecules (sterols). For a long time scientists thought that seafood elevates cholesterol levels or would be harmful to those with cholesterol blockage that cause heart attack or stroke. In fact, seafood-only diets will lower cholesterol in most patients, often dramatically. You and your physician can test this yourselves by measuring cholesterol levels at the end of Food Phase 1 and again at the end of Food Phase 2.

Toxins — But what about the mercury and other toxins reportedly found in seafood? Magazine articles have noted mercury, cadmium, and dioxin (PCBs) found in different fish populations. However, levels are usually present at concentrations that are medically insignificant. Only farm-raised salmon from Europe have been found with PCB levels that could be a risk if you ate it daily for years or decades. European fish are raised with bait fish caught in more polluted waters of the North and Baltic Seas. Toxin levels are not significant for North or South American farm-raised salmon. Check with your local Fish and Wildlife Department regarding fish caught in local streams. Most states check toxin levels in local seafood.

Bacteria are present in some shellfish, especially oysters and clams. Vibrio species of bacteria are common in salt marshes and are not contaminants, but rather, normal marsh inhabitants. Raw shellfish might contain sufficient numbers of bacteria to cause

Avoid eating raw seafood if you have liver or immune disease, you are being treated with chemotherapy, or if you take antacid medication.

⌒ *Section B: Diving In...* ⌒

IMPOSSIBLE TO GAIN ON SEAFOOD

The average woman requires 11 calories/pound/day to maintain weight; the average man requires 12 calories/pound/day. Those numbers represent your Basal Metabolic Rate (BMR).

Subtract one calorie/pound/day from your total metabolism at age 40 and again at age 65 since metabolism naturally slows with age. Using these calculations, consider the following example:

To gain one pound of fat, a 160-pound, 40 year-old woman would need to consume 5,100 calories. Of those calories, 1,600 could be for maintenance (10 calories/day X 160 pounds = BMR) and 3,500 would represent the energy needed for one pound of fat.

That means, she would need to eat 13 pounds of seafood (5,100 calories divided by 400 calories/pound) to gain one pound in a given day! She would need to eat 5 pounds per day to gain one pound in a week.

Not likely!

symptoms (diarrhea). Individuals with liver or immune disease (on chemotherapy) should not eat raw seafood. Those taking antacid medication should also avoid raw shellfish, as stomach acid kills most bacteria inhabiting shellfish. Except for steaming, all other forms of cooking destroy the bacteria. A few cases of bacterial dysentery have been reported in steamed lobsters. Horseradish used to dip raw oysters has been shown to kill shellfish bacteria. Shellfish-related diarrhea is rare.

SEAFOOD AND CALORIES

Seafood is the best calorie "bang for your buck" at 25 calories per ounce (35 per ounce for fatty fishes). This means that one pound (16 ounces) of seafood is only 400 calories if cooked without fat or oil. Since you would have to eat more calories than you burn to gain weight, it is virtually impossible to gain weight on non-fried or non-sautéed seafood.

CATEGORIES OF SEAFOOD — ARE THERE DIFFERENCES?

Are there nutritional and caloric differences between types of seafood? What about shellfish vs. fish? Yes there are differences, but practically speaking, the differences are not significant enough to cause concern. Fatty fish are higher in Omega 3 fats and have slightly more calories. These few extra calories are insignificant to weight gain and may be offset by health benefits. We recommend using seafood in Food Phase 2 because seafood tastes great, is filling, has few calories per serving, and contains no nutrients that induce abnormal chemistry.

Variety is important to keep interest, prevent boredom, or cause aversion. Using different types of seafood in Food Phase 2 will likely make seafood more desirable. Experiment!

What if I Can't or Won't Eat seafood?

If you are allergic to seafood, you may use poultry or vegetables in Phase 2. Or, you can substitute nonfat cottage cheese. Be sure to read the directions for Food Phase 3 (Poultry) or Food Phase 4 (Vegetables) or Food Phase 12 (Dairy) before you begin.

Methods of Cooking Seafood

Seafood meat is flaky and porous compared to a steak. You can break off little pieces of cooked fish with a fork, which you could not do with a piece of steak. This means that the meat fibers of fish are able to soak up oil. In fact, fish cooked in oil or butter will soak up enough oil to equal the same caloric value of fatty red meat. Red meat on the other hand is already saturated with fat and therefore cannot soak up additional oil.

With these facts in mind, you'll want to avoid fried or sautéed fish (unless used as a "splurge" meal). Instead, prepare your seafood boiled, poached, broiled, steamed, baked, or grilled. The PrescriptFit™ recipes

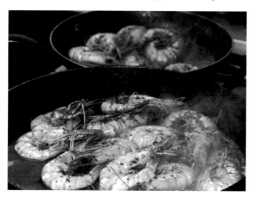

Vegetarian? No problem. Simply skip the seafood, poultry, meat, and pork Phases. Remember, the PrescriptFit™ product, with a multivitamin is PERFECT food. Everything else is entertainment.

Fried or sautéed seafood contains 125 calories/ounce compared to 25 calories/ounce for seafood prepared without oil. The extra 100 calories/ounce is totally from the oil. (Oil contains 125 calories/level tablespoon). Remember that one-mile of walking burns 100 calories. Therefore, frying and sautéing seafood requires one mile of walking to pay for the calories in only one ounce of fried seafood.

❧ *Section B: Diving In...* ❧

TIPS/HINTS FOR COOKING SEAFOOD

1. If you're not a fan of "fishy tasting" fish, try adding lemon juice, parsley, green onion tops, and capers.

2. Always rinse your seafood before cooking.

3. Do not overcook. If your seafood is tough or rubbery, you have overcooked it. Most seafood only takes around 5–8 minutes to cook on the stove; 12–20 minutes in the oven.

4. Add ½ cup of chicken broth and 1 tablespoon of butter powder when cooking pan-seared seafood to make a light and delicious sauce.

5. In Food Phases 2, 3, and 4, try mixing PrescriptFit™ soups with vegetables or meats to make stews or casserole dishes.

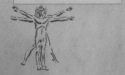

will help you use stocks and flavorings to achieve better flavor from sautéed fish .

The most common "mistake" when preparing flavorful seafood is over cooking. You needn't worry about cooking fish to a "safe" temperature since raw fish is safe to eat (if fresh). Fatty fish is especially vulnerable to over cooking. The oil in the fish changes flavor when it is heated. Therefore, cooked tuna or salmon tastes radically different than slightly browned fish with a pink center.

Shopping for Seafood

Often, people are wary of buying seafood simply because they don't know what to buy or what to look for. Here are some simple tips:

1. Buy fresh from a fish market if possible.

2. If you buy from a supermarket, buy frozen fish. Do not buy the fish from a display case. The seafood is almost always previously frozen and thawed in the store unless it is specifically marked "fresh caught."

3. When buying frozen seafood, buy sealed bags. Look for bags with little or no ice crystals in the bag.

4. Thaw the fish, in its bag, in a bowl of room temperature water. Rinse the fish once thawed. It is then ready to cook.

Use shopping to reinforce your Food Phase strategies. If you buy seafood from the supermarket, go directly to the seafood section when beginning your shopping, since seafood is the first "food" Phase of the PrescriptFit™ Plan. From the seafood section, go directly to poultry (Food Phase 3), then vegetables (Food Phase 4). Strategic shopping will reinforce strategic diet planning.

Although there are no restrictions on the amount of seafood you eat, several ingredients commonly used when preparing seafood are excluded from Phase 2, including flour, cornmeal, bread crumbs, and most store-bought batter. Nevertheless, you'll discover numerous simple and delicious methods for preparing seafood that allow you to enjoy what you are eating without foregoing taste.

Listed at right are all of the ingredients needed for the recipes in Phase 2. These are divided into "staples," which you'll want in your cupboard for later Food Phases, and Phase 2 ingredients (see pages 78–79). Also included are optional ingredients that you may use to experiment with your particular palette. You may choose to add similar ingredients or additives that do not appear on the list below.

You will notice that several herbs and fresh garlic are used to season the dishes. These ingredients are approved for this phase as a seasoning. Feel free to experiment; just remember that all flavor additives must meet the requirement of being sugar-free and fat-free. Many of the ingredients will be used again in the Phase 3.

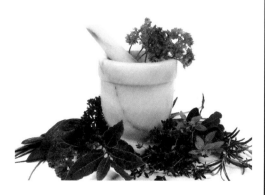

THE GROCERY LIST

STAPLES

- Chicken broth or chicken bouillon cubes (soft variety preferred)
- Fat-free butter spray or Benecol® spread
- Butter powder (Butter Buds® or Molly McButter® powder found in the seasoning aisle)
- Black pepper
- Salt
- Cajun/Creole seasoning mix or red pepper seasoning mix
- Blackening seasoning (If available)
- Non-stick cooking spray
- Garlic powder
- Balsamic Vinegar
- Worcestershire sauce
- Tony Chachere's™ seasoning mix

Continued...

The Amino Solution
©2009 Stanford A. Owen, MD

THE GROCERY LIST

PHASE 2 INGREDIENTS

- White-type fish filets (white fish, catfish, tilapia, etc.)
- Shrimp (fresh or frozen)
- Salmon steaks
- 1 fresh tuna steak (may substitute salmon)
- 1 tablespoon beef broth (use chicken broth if substituting salmon)
- Fresh rosemary (may substitute dried rosemary)
- Fresh sage (may substitute dried sage)
- Fresh dill (may substitute dried dill)
- Lemons or lemon juice (fresh lemon juice highly suggested)
- Chopped or minced garlic
- Chives or green onions
- Parsley

Continued...

BOB OWEN'S SEAFOOD RECIPES

SKILLET LEMON FISH

2–3 filets white type fish (white fish, catfish, tilapia, etc.)
1 scoop PrescriptFit™ Chicken Soup, mixed with ½ cup water
1–2 teaspoons Creole/Cajun seasoning mix or black pepper
½ cup chicken broth
1–2 tablespoons lemon juice
1 tablespoon fat-free butter spray or Benecol® butter
1 teaspoon of Butter Buds® powder or Molly McButter® powder seasoning
Non-stick cooking spray

Lightly coat a large sauté pan with non-stick cooking spray and heat to medium-high. Rinse fish filets in cold water. Pat dry with a paper towel. Mix the PrescriptFit™ Chicken Soup and water together until all lumps are dissolved. Add pepper or seasoning mix, then place in a shallow bowl. Dip the fish into the soup batter and place in the pre-heated pan.

Cook the fish on one side for 2–4 minutes, then flip and cook for an additional 2–5 minutes or until fully cooked. Spray non-stick spray, if needed, on dry sections of the batter.

Remove the fish and set it aside. Add the broth, butter spray or Benecol Butter, butter powder, and lemon juice to the pan, scraping any remains from the bottom.

Cook for 2–4 minutes on medium-high. Drizzle the sauce over the fish. Add salt and enjoy.

DEVON — NEW WAYS TO ENJOY SEAFOOD

CASE STUDY

Devon grew up in the Mississippi Delta. She never ate seafood that was not fried. The thought of baked fish made her nauseated. Her usual experience with poultry was either fried by her grandmother, or usually, from a fast food establishment. Even the Thanksgiving turkey is fried and injected with butter.

Willing to keep an open mind, Devon's husband started preparing seafood on the barbecue pit. They then experimented with PrescriptFit recipes (some of which have been used in a national television cooking program). Over a period of several years, both Devon and her husband became fans of PrescriptFit food preparation. They still eat fried foods but on "splurge" meals twice a week or less.

LEMON GARLIC SHRIMP

1 pound of shrimp (peeled)
2 tablespoons chopped or minced garlic
½ cup chicken stock
1–2 tablespoons lemon juice
2 teaspoons Benecol Butter or fat free butter spray
1 tablespoon butter powder
1 tablespoon chives or green onions (chopped)
1 tablespoon parsley (chopped)
1 teaspoon black pepper
Salt to desired taste
1–2 dashes of red pepper or Cajun/Creole seasoning mix
Non-stick cooking spray

Lightly coat a saucepan with non-stick cooking spray. Heat to med-high. Season the

THE GROCERY LIST

OPTIONAL INGREDIENTS

- Thyme
- Oregano
- Basil
- Chili powder
- Capers
- Cilantro
- Bay leaves
- Leeks
- White pepper
- Crushed red peppers
- Jalapeño peppers
- Sea salt
- Kosher salt

shrimp with red pepper or Cajun/Creole seasoning, salt, and black pepper. Add the shrimp and the chopped garlic to the saucepan. Cook for 2–4 minutes, flipping the shrimp at least once. Do not let the garlic brown. Immediately, add the chicken stock. Cook the broth until the mixture begins to thicken. Add the remaining ingredients. Squeeze the lemon juice and add 1–4 teaspoons to taste. Finish with green onions, salt, black pepper, and parsley.

SEARED WHITE FISH

2–3 filets white fish (tilapia, white fish or catfish; or substitute peeled shrimp)
Blackening seasoning (may substitute Cajun/Creole seasoning, black pepper, or red pepper)
Salt
Lemon juice
Non-stick cooking spray or 1 tablespoon Benecol® Spread

Coat the fish filets or shrimp with seasoning mix. Lightly coat each side of the filets with non-stick cooking spray. Spray a very small amount of non-stick spray into a skillet or sauté pan, or melt the Benecol® Spread. Heat on med-high until the pan begins smoking. Sear both sides of the fish in the skillet for 1–2 minutes on each side or until the fish is cooked to a desired preference.

Remove the fish. Add salt and drizzle with lemon juice to taste.

Baked Black Pepper Fish or Shrimp

2–3 filets of white fish (tilapia, white fish or
  catfish) or peeled shrimp (tail on or off)
Black pepper (cracked black pepper or
  Malabar pepper preferred)
Salt
Lemon juice
Non-stick cooking spray

Preheat oven to 375 degrees. Lightly coat a
baking pan or dish with non-stick cooking
spray. Place filets or shrimp face up on the
pan. Sprinkle with black pepper and salt. Bake
fish for 12–18 minutes or until fish is cooked to
your desired preference. Once cooked, drizzle
with lemon juice.

Dill, Rosemary & Sage Salmon

1–2 salmon steaks
2 cups chicken broth or 1 dose PrescriptFit™
  Chicken Soup
1 tablespoon fat-free butter spray
1 tablespoon lemon juice
2 stalks fresh rosemary (may substitute with
  1 teaspoon dried rosemary)
1 tablespoon fresh dill, minced (may
  substitute with 1 teaspoon dried dill)
8 leaves fresh sage (may substitute with 1
  teaspoon of dried sage)
½ – 1 teaspoon of black pepper
½ – 1 teaspoon of Cajun/Creole seasoning
Salt to taste

Heat the chicken broth on high in a large
saucepan until boiling. Reduce heat to
medium. Add the seasonings to the broth.
Rinse salmon steaks in cold water. Place in
simmering broth for two minutes. Flip the fish
with a spatula then continue to simmer for 2–5
minutes until the fish is cooked on both sides

to taste. Carefully remove the salmon and set to the side. Chop rosemary leaves (begin at the tip and cut in small pieces. Roll Sage leaves lengthwise and cut into 4–6 slices. Add all ingredients to the broth except the lemon. Cook for 3–5 minutes until the sauce begins to thicken. Add lemon juice. Drizzle over the top of the fish.

Cracked Black Pepper Seared Tuna Steak

- 1 fresh tuna steak (may substitute salmon)
- 1 tablespoon cracked black pepper or Malabar Black Pepper
- 1 teaspoon salt
- Non-stick cooking spray
- 1 teaspoon lemon juice
- 1 tablespoon beef broth (use chicken broth if substituting salmon)

Lightly coat a non-stick sauté pan with non-stick cooking spray. Rinse the tuna steak with cold water. Rub the tuna steak with the salt and pepper until thoroughly coated. Heat the pan to medium-high. Sear the tuna in the pan for three minutes on each side.

To serve medium-rare: Remove the tuna steak from the pan and set to the side. Add remaining ingredients to the pan. Reduce the mixture and drizzle over the tuna.

To serve medium to medium-well: Do not remove from pan. Add remaining ingredients and cook until the desired temperature

Important: Tuna will taste dry and lose flavor if overcooked. If fresh, the tuna is best at medium to medium rare.

PHASE 3 POULTRY

Poultry is your next logical addition to the PrescriptFit™ MNT Plan because, like seafood, poultry is inexpensive, filling, low in calories, versatile, tastes great, and does not provoke cytokine production. Though you may choose to substitute poultry for seafood, poultry typically follows seafood since the fat content is higher and, therefore, the calorie content is higher.

POULTRY AS NUTRITION

Poultry contains no carbohydrate. Poultry muscle is quite lean, containing minimal amounts of fat. Most of the fat content of poultry, which is saturated, harmful fat, is contained in the skin on the surface of the muscle. Both the skin and surface fat should be removed before cooking.

Poultry contains about 50 calories/ounce (seafood is 25 calories/ounce) due to the increased fat content. Leaving the skin on brings the calorie/ounce to about 75–100, depending on how much drainage is allowed during cooking. An average breast weighs about 4 ounces, or 200 calories without the skin. Leaving the skin on not only raises the

Reminder:
- Continue 6–8 or more PrescriptFit™ amino acid doses per day.
- Use PrescriptFit™ shakes or soups before or with meals.
- Use foods from Phases 2 and 3.
- Take a multi-vitamin supplement.
- Drink 5 cups of water or calorie-free beverage daily.

Dosing:
No portion or dose restrictions are used for poultry. All you can eat. Enjoy!

Phase 3: Poultry

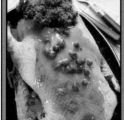
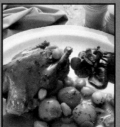
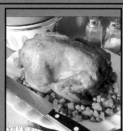

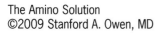

☞ Section B: Diving In... ☜

Remember, saturated fat provokes cytokines!

calorie count to around 300–400 calories, it also adds saturated fat, which provokes cytokines along with adverse effects on insulin, cortisone, and lipid (cholesterol) metabolism.

Poultry protein is high in the amino acid tryptophan. Tryptophan can cause sedation and may be responsible for the "coma" or excessive tired feeling that follows a typical Thanksgiving meal of turkey. However, by Food Phase 3 most people are feeling so much more energized that any sedating effect from poultry is minimal. Do be on the lookout for sedating effects that become uncomfortable. If excessive sedation is a problem, use poultry sparingly.

As with any meat, poultry is filling and satiating. The protein takes longer to digest

SAM — FINDING A WORKING BALANCE

Sam had been diagnosed with sleep apnea, severe fatigue, and high blood pressure when he began the PrescriptFit™ MNT Plan. He became symptom-free (no fatigue), abolished snoring, and normalized blood pressure without medication after completing Food Phase 2 (seafood + amino acids) of the Plan (4 weeks). Within one week of adding Food Phase 3 (poultry), his wife noticed increased snoring, and Sam reported fatigue to a level one-half his initial experience.

He admitted using large amounts of poultry and minimal seafood the first week into Food Phase 3. I had him return to Food Phase 2 for one week, then resume Food Phase 3 with limited amounts (one meal/day) of poultry. His snoring and fatigue completely resolved when he resumed Food Phase 2 and did not return with the limited poultry when re-starting Food Phase 3.

Sam had no further problems with Food Phase 4 (vegetables) or beyond.

CASE STUDY

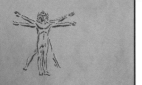

and does not vigorously stimulate insulin unless a large amount of chicken fat is consumed. Like seafood, poultry is deficient in certain vitamins. Continuation of a multivitamin is mandatory.

Poultry Toxin Myths

The U.S. Food and Drug Administration has scrutinized poultry producers for the commercial use of artificial hormones and phosphates to enhance growth. No definite link to human disease has been documented. Most modern poultry farms do not add toxic products to the feed, and many progressive growing houses are using natural feed devoid of hormones or growth-producing nutrients.

"Free Range" chicken is very lean and tastes different from commercially raised chicken. Range-fed chickens can quit feeding when they are not hungry or when the work of finding food is more uncomfortable than the hunger. Chickens confined to a small space in a chicken factory cannot move (exercise), are bored (no "playground" interaction), and are constantly exposed to high fat feed. No wonder they are fatter than range chickens! Sound familiar to human obesity? Range chicken is preferable if available and affordable.

Categories of Poultry — Chicken, Turkey, Duck, Quail, Pheasant, Other Birds

There are differences between different birds and differences among same bird species depending on how the birds are raised and fed (keep in mind human analogies). All birds fed "naturally" are leaner and contain less fat.

"Free Range" chicken is a term used to describe chicken raised "the old fashioned way" in the barnyard or fields, either pecking a meal from grass seeds or being fed grain by the local farmer.

The Amino Solution
©2009 Stanford A. Owen, MD

Section B: Diving In... ॐ

CALORIES & POULTRY

Poultry contains 50 calories per ounce or twice as many calories as seafood due to fat content of the skin and meat.

Still quite a calorie bargain, one can eat a pound of poultry for only 800 calories. A generous 8-ounce serving is only 400 calories.

Using the 40-year-old, 160-pound female with a BMR of 10 calories/pound/day to maintain weight, two pounds of poultry/day (800 calories per pound = 1600 calories) would be necessary to maintain weight with no other calorie intake.

To gain a pound a day (3500 calories over 1600 calories or 5100 calories) she would have to eat 6 pounds of poultry/day!

To gain one pound over an entire week, or 2100 calories for seven days, the 40-year-old female would have to consume almost 3 pounds of poultry per day — not likely!

"Naturally" means as they would feed and exercise in nature: searching for food; finding only lean food; resting when full; running from enemies; chasing mates; and defending territory from intruders. Imagine how much easier to keep your weight under control if you live "naturally!"

Duck is most capable of accumulating fat when fed excessively. Therefore, domestic duck is quite high in calories (100 calories/ounce unless stripped completely of fat). If you ever roast duck, you will notice a large puddle of grease in the pot after cooking. Wild duck is nonfat, even with the skin, and tastes nothing like domestic duck. Wild duck requires prolonged cooking with many herbs (see recipes) for palatability.

Chicken is next most fat. Turkey is quite lean. Since turkeys are difficult to keep penned in confined space like chickens, they get some exercise.

Pheasant and quail are quite lean, especially if wild. Ostrich and emus are large birds that are raised commercially but have not caught on as inexpensive food sources. These two birds are quite lean for the same reasons as turkey—they are too large to confine and must be "range" fed. No exercise with food in front of your face at all times keeps birds fat—just like humans!

SAFELY STORING POULTRY

As you may know, poultry is easily contaminated with bacteria. As with humans, animals kept in a confined space with common handlers spread germs by proximity. At slaughter, these bacteria are transmitted through fecal material. Salmonella, the most common organism found contaminating poultry, causes intestinal disease with diarrhea. Careless handling of intestine in the butchering process can spread the disease. Some studies found 40 percent of chicken meat tested positive for salmonella. While community rates of diarrhea are lower than 40 percent, play it safe and assume your meat is contaminated. Poison-producing E. coli bacteria also has been found in chicken. Here are some tips for safely handling poultry:

- Always store poultry in the refrigerator until ready to cook.

- Thaw frozen poultry in the refrigerator or in the microwave just before cooking.

- Don't eat undercooked poultry! Use a meat thermometer, and make sure it registers 180 degrees (170 degrees for breast meat) before you stop cooking it.

There are no restrictions on the amount of poultry you eat. However, several ingredients commonly used when preparing poultry are excluded from Phase 3, including flour, cornmeal, bread crumbs and most store-bought batter. Furthermore, you must remove the skin and visible fat before cooking your poultry. You'll find many appealing ways to prepare poultry without adding a lot of calories and fat!

The grocery list, on the next page, includes the ingredients you'll need for the recipes in this Phase. You may also use the "Optional Ingredients" from the list in Phase 2 (page 79). You may choose to add similar ingredients or additives that do not appear on the grocery list. Feel free to experiment; just remember that all flavor additives must be sugar-free and fat-free additions.

The most important aspect of the PrescriptFit™ MNT program is the amino acid supplement. Make sure that you are consuming the correct amount of doses for your plan.

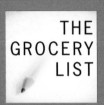

THE GROCERY LIST

Staples from Phase 2 PLUS: Chicken (boneless or bone-in, skinless, whole or cut up, depending on recipe)

- Optional: PrescriptFit™ Chicken Soup for gravy
- Beef broth
- Chicken broth
- One onion
- Thyme (dried or fresh)
- Fresh or dried sage
- Lemons or fresh lemon juice
- Chopped, minced or cloves of garlic
- Chives or green onions
- Parsley

If you're dreaming of crispy, greasy, fried chicken, wake up! No fried foods are allowed, except for "splurge" meals, during the PrescriptFit™ MNT Plan. Like fish, poultry meat is more porous and "stringy" than beef and can accumulate oil when frying or basting in its own grease. Like fish, poultry will accumulate enough oil when fried to equal caloric content of beef at 125 calories/ounce, over twice the calories as non-fried poultry prepared without the skin (grilled, baked, broiled, boiled, or stewed in broth).

If you're one who craves fried chicken, save it for one of your eight "splurge" meals per month allowed in Food Phase 9 and beyond.

You'll discover delicious, new ways to prepare poultry. Poultry makes excellent soups with relative ease by combining chicken broth and chicken bouillon cubes, which taste similar to a homemade stock. You can also make gravy by combining broth, bouillon and PrescriptFit™ Chicken Soup. Finally, anyone can make a low-fat, low-calorie butter flavor sauce by combining chicken broth, bouillon and butter flavored powder, such as Butter Buds® or Molly McButter®.

Because poultry is a popular source of protein throughout the world, there are many styles of cooking poultry. You may want to experiment with regional flavor combinations to develop a distinctive dish. For example, if you want to make Italian style chicken, use typical Italian ingredients such as basil, oregano, thyme, sage, and garlic. Or, if you want to cook a Cajun style dish, use red and black pepper, garlic, onion powder, celery salt, etc. All seasonings are acceptable as long as they do not add sugar or fat to the recipe.

CHARLEY AND HIS WIFE — THEIR AMINO SOLUTION

Charley is a meat eater. He could eat meat or follow the Atkins diet forever. His wife, on the other hand, hates meat. She is borderline vegetarian and loves pasta. Charley blames his wife's pasta and bread on his beer-belly physique. The two compromised: Charley would use the barbecue grill as often as possible to prepare seafood, poultry, and meat dishes while grilling vegetables. He was responsible for being creative with the veggies. Much to his surprise (and his wife's), Charley became enthralled with vegetable and meat dishes.

It soon became apparent that, indeed, his wife's addiction to carbs was an issue. Since they agreed to "splurging" two meals per week, she was forced to consider other carb-like foods.

She focused on dessert dishes made with PrescriptFit™ products and snack bars to make up the sweet/carb cravings. He remained a meat-a-holic with a vegetarian flare. While their basic food instincts were not changed (they rarely do), their style developed individual characteristics. Most marriage weight gain is similar to Charley and his wife: trying to "eat together" with different preferences and styles—a sure path to weight gain.

BOB OWEN'S POULTRY RECIPES

CHICKEN SOUP

2 large chicken breasts — skinned, boneless
    or bone-in
3 cups chicken broth
1 large bouillon cube mixed with
    1 cup water
1–2 large leeks – sliced
1 tablespoon dried or fresh thyme
1 bay leaf
1 teaspoon sage
1–2 tablespoons minced parsley
1 tablespoon chopped green onions
1 teaspoon cajun/creole seasoning mix
Black pepper & salt
1 scoop PrescriptFit™ Chicken Soup

As a rule, poultry is much more tender if cooked in a broth, gravy, or stew than if cooked on a grill or dry in an oven. Nevertheless, low heat, slow cooking, or slow smoking is a fantastic means of retaining the tenderness of the poultry while adding flavor. Just be sure to monitor for tenderness while cooking.

☞ *Section B: Diving In...* ☜

Season chicken with seasoning mix & black pepper. In a stock pot, add remaining ingredients except for PrescriptFit™ and bring to a boil. Reduce heat and simmer for 20–30 minutes. Dissolve PrescriptFit™ in the mixture and stir until thick; finish with parsley and green onions. Remove chicken, cut into cubes/small pieces, then add pieces back into the soup. Serve at once.

Baked Chicken (Pieces)

Chicken pieces (skinless, cut up)
Cajun/Creole seasoning mix
Black pepper & salt

Preheat oven to 375 degrees. Place chicken pieces on a baking sheet. Dust the outside of the chicken with Cajun/Creole seasoning mix, black pepper, and salt. Rub seasonings into the meat. Place in oven and cook for 25–30 minutes or until the outside of the chicken begins to brown. Serve.

Baked Chicken (Whole)

1 whole chicken
1 onion peeled and quartered
3–6 cloves of garlic, cut in half
2 cups chicken broth
Black pepper & salt

Preheat oven to 375 degrees. Remove skin from the chicken and discard. Remove all parts from the cavity of the chicken. Wash chicken. Stuff the cavity of the chicken with the onion and the garlic. Dust chicken with black pepper and salt. Place breast side down in a deep baking dish or pan. Pour broth into the bottom of the pan. Bake for 20–30 minutes, then flip the chicken over and continue to cook for 25–35 minutes until the entire chicken is cooked thoroughly. Baste chicken with broth every 15 minutes. Add 2–3 tablespoons of PrescriptFit™ Chicken Soup Mix for thick gravy. Carve and serve.

My best advice for your poultry experiments: Don't limit your options. Yet, until you become familiar with new seasonings, you'd be wise to add small amounts of seasoning at a time. This is especially true of the more pungent herbs, such as cilantro, anise or fennel seed, or spices like red or white pepper.

BLACKENED CHICKEN

> 1–2 boneless/skinless chicken breasts
> Non-stick, butter-flavored cooking spray or
>   Benecol® Spread
> Blackening or Cajun/Creole seasoning

Dust chicken with peppers until evenly covered on both sides. Rub seasoning into the chicken. Spray non-stick spray or melt Benecol® Spread evenly to cover the bottom of the skillet. Heat on highest setting until smoke readily appears from the pan. Simultaneously place both chicken breasts in the pan. Cook at least 20 seconds or until blackening occurs. Flip and repeat. Remove pan from heat and allow to cool. Add two tablespoons of water or chicken broth , cover, and cook on medium heat until done (depends on type of stove).

BRAISED GARLIC AND GREEN ONION CHICKEN

> Skinless chicken with or without bone
> 5–7 chopped green onions
> 2 tablespoons chopped garlic
> 1 lemon (optional)
> Cajun/Creole seasoning mix
> Black pepper & salt
> 1 cup chicken broth or bouillon
> (Optional) 1 scoop PrescriptFit™ Chicken
>   Soup mixed with ¾ cup of water
> Non-stick cooking spray or Benecol® Spread

Dust the chicken with Cajun/Creole seasoning mix, black pepper, and salt. Lightly coat a sauté pan with non-stick cooking spray or Benecol® Spread. Heat to med-high; then place the dusted chicken into the pan. Cook on both sides until brown. Once brown on both sides, add chopped garlic and green onions. Cook for 5 minutes, taking care not to burn the garlic. Add chicken broth (or the optional pre-mixed PrescriptFit™ Chicken Soup). Cover and cook for 10–15 minutes on med-low heat.

Always use a meat thermometer to ensure meat is 180 degrees.

Optional: Stir lemon juice into the sauce for Lemon Chicken.

The Amino Solution
©2009 Stanford A. Owen, MD

⪢ Section B: Diving In... ⪡

PHASE 4 VEGETABLES

Vegetables are added to the early phases of the PrescriptFit™ MNT Plan because they are low in calories and simple sugar and high in filling fiber. They are also loaded with vitamins, minerals, antioxidants, and phytonutrients.

VEGETABLES AS NUTRITION

Vegetables enhance blood vessel function, fight cancer, and balance intestinal bacteria colonies. Vegetables can be used to enhance the flavor of the amino acid supplements as well as the seafood and chicken recipes from Food Phases 2–3. Vegetables provide an endless variety of color, texture, smell, taste, and nutrition. Vegetables are filling.

Unlimited amounts of vegetables on the Phase 4 list are allowed in Food Phase 4 of the PrescriptFit™ MNT Plan. However, starchy vegetables (corn, potatoes, peas, dried beans, winter squash) are reserved for Food Phase 13. The larger carbohydrate load added by starchy vegetables could induce insulin resistance, cause a relapse of symptoms, and promote weight gain. If you crave starchy vegetables, you'll be better off saving them for a splurge meal after you've achieved significant improvement and weight loss.

Phase 4: Vegetables

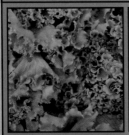
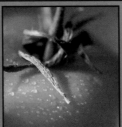
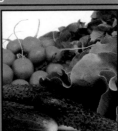

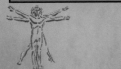

Food Phase 4 of the PrescriptFit™ MNT plan recommends five or more servings of vegetables per day, along with 6–8 doses of amino acids, and as much

Dosing: There is no portion or dose restriction with non-starchy vegetables. Eat as much as you desire—the more the better.

seafood or poultry as desired. At the very least, include a vegetable serving at breakfast, lunch, and supper. If you combine two servings at lunch and dinner with one serving for breakfast, you'll meet your five-a-day requirement.

VEGETABLE MYTHS

Many people are convinced that consumption of vegetable extracts, squeezed vegetable juices, and huge doses of vitamins will bring health or prevent disease. The public buys and consumes these products every day at staggering costs, never suspecting there is a better, safer, less-expensive way to enjoy the benefits of vegetables.

Most of the benefits of herbal products were extrapolated from the evidence that people consuming diets very high in vegetable content were spared many chronic illnesses associated with obesity. Whole vegetables (and fruit) behave much differently in the human intestine than juiced, dried, or concentrated portions of those vegetables. Bacteria in the intestine grow on vegetable fiber, vegetable nutrients, and vegetable sugars. The bacteria produce chemicals that increase anticancer immune function. By using purified products, the benefits of whole vegetables might well be missed.

Remember — variety prevents boredom. You've read this over and over in this book; it should be your mantra by now!

Eating five servings or more of diverse vegetables per day assures vitamin, mineral, and intestinal bacterial balance. An ideal strategy is to consume five different colors of vegetables daily: green, yellow, purple, red, or orange. Each color:

- Represents different phytonutrients, vitamins, minerals, and plant sugars.

- Adds different flavor and variety

ORGANIC VEGETABLES

Debate has raged for years over the health implications of organically grown vegetables versus traditional commercial farming methods. "Organic" vegetables are grown without pesticide, without artificial growth-enhancing chemicals or fertilizers, and are not shipped with preservative chemicals. Proponents claim organic vegetables contain more minerals, vitamins, and nutrients.

In more than 20 years of practicing medicine, I have yet to directly diagnose, or contribute a death, to pesticides found in commercially grown produce. However, every day I meet a new patient who suffers from a fatal disease directly caused by fat and calories.

Buy organic produce if you prefer. But, keep in mind that your food choices should be realistic and truly pertinent to your health; avoiding vegetables because organic options are either not available or are more expensive probably isn't a healthy food choice.

CALORIES & VEGETABLE CATEGORIES

Vegetables, including starchy vegetables, are the lowest calorie food per unit of any food group. Vegetables are even lower in calories, by weight, than seafood. This is because vegetables are high in non-digestible fiber and low in sugar. Vegetables are bulky and filling.

We measure vegetables by the cup. To visualize one cup, try this experiment: chop any type of vegetable, place into a measuring cup, then pour the contents onto a dinner plate. Note the large volume on the dinner plate. Make a mental note how few calories per cup fill up that plate.

Vegetables differ in calorie content by the amount of carbohydrate, fat, and fiber they contain. Most vegetables have relatively small amounts of fat or protein. Green, leafy vegetables are very low in calories, while starchy vegetables (corn, dried beans, potatoes) have the highest caloric content – 200 calories per cup. One cup of beans will almost cover a dinner plate; yet it contains less calories than two bites of a fatty steak.

While not all vegetables are listed on page 96, visualize which category a vegetable might fit if not listed. For example: is asparagus more like leafy greens and broccoli or more like corn? While asparagus is crunchy like both groups, there is no such thing as asparagus oil. Asparagus will fit the lower calorie group. Vegetables are so low in calories, you can't make a big mistake, even with starchy vegetables.

The table on the next page features the main vegetable categories by calorie. Remember, for any food, you must walk one mile at 100 calories per mile to "pay back" calories. Is your choice worth the calories?

PEGGY — GETTING WELL & SAVING MONEY

I recently examined a 220-pound diabetic woman taking 20 different herbal and vitamin supplements per day, spending huge amounts of time on the Internet researching herb science, and feeling miserable with out-of-control diabetes and hypertension.

I discontinued all her herbs, saving her over $400 dollars per month, preventing unknown drug interactions, and simplifying her day immensely. She felt fantastic and gained perfect control of her diabetes and hypertension after only Food Phase 1 of the high risk (14-day) PrescriptFit™ MNT Plan, consuming only PrescriptFit amino acid shakes and soups and a single multiple vitamin.

She completed two sessions of the 13-Phase Plan and never needed medication again. She lost 80 pounds and returned to a full life. Her medication and herb bill dropped from $1,200/month to zero! I see similar cases every day in my clinic.

CASE STUDY

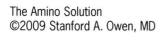

⌘ Section B: Diving In... ⌘

Vegetable	Calories/cup*	Amount of Vegetable equivalent to 1 bite of steak
Lettuce, Spinach, Turnip Greens, Cucumbers, Celery	10	10 cups
Bell Pepper, Celery, Summer Squash (yellow)	20	5 cups
Carrots, Asparagus, Okra, Green Beans, Cauliflower, Broccoli, Tomatoes	40	3 cups
Onions	60	2 cups
Eggplant, Cabbage, and Brussel Sprouts	20	5 cups

These calorie contents are based on fresh preparation without condiments

Though the vegetables listed below are a great caloric value compared to other food categories, they are higher in sugar and starch. Save these until Phase 13.

Vegetable	Calories/cup*	Amt of Vegetable equivalent to 1 bite of steak
Winter Squash (Hubbard, Butternut, Scorn), Stewed Tomatoes	80	1.5 cups
Fresh Peas. Fresh Beans, Diced Potatoes	120	1 cup
Corn, Mashed Potatoes	140	1 cup
Dried Beans/Peas	200	1 cup = 4 bites of steak or 2 miles of walking

These calorie contents are based on fresh preparation without condiments

Shopping for Vegetables

Spend most of your grocery store time in the vegetable section, heading there right after seafood and poultry to reinforce Food Phase thinking. This is where you'll want to do the most planning since there so many varieties and potential combinations exist. Experiment with at least one new vegetable weekly. After shopping the fresh vegetable section, go directly to the canned or dried vegetable section to supplement your variety.

Look for condiments low in calories for dipping or mixing vegetables for salads. Avoid butter, cheese, and salad dressings with sugar or fat. Avoid any dressing over 20 calories / tablespoon. PrescriptFit salad dressing recipes contain less than 10 calories / tablespoon.

Cooking & Seasoning Vegetables

A good way to eat your five servings of vegetables is to chop them and add to PrescriptFit Beef or Chicken soups. Broths are an excellent way to enhance vegetable flavor and variety without adding calories. Soups make excellent gravy when mixed thickly.

Baking or broiling vegetables also bring out vegetable flavor without soaking them in oil or butter. Chop up a variety of vegetables of different colors in about one-inch pieces. Place vegetables in a pan and spray with vegetable oil or butter spray (PAM™ has a nice selection). Broil the vegetables in the oven until slightly brown; sprinkling your favorite seasoning (ours is Paul Prudhomme's Magic Seasoning™ at www.chefpaul.com). Combining squash, asparagus, onion, bell pepper, and eggplant gets all the colors in a single, delicious dish.

Raw vegetables are the most nutritious method of consuming vegetables. Leave raw vegetables displayed around the house and bring snack trays of vegetables and fruit to work.

Canned vegetables are equal in calories to fresh vegetables unless prepared with sugars or stew meats. Read the contents label on canned vegetables. They are mostly accurate.

If you like butter flavor, use Benecol® or Smart Balance™ spread made from plant stanols. These products lower cholesterol and triglycerides almost as much as cholesterol medication and improve artery function. They also taste great.

Enhance the flavor of your vegetables with PrescriptFit™ Chicken or Beef Soup.

The Amino Solution
©2009 Stanford A. Owen, MD

⌐ *Section B: Diving In...* ⌐

Bob Owen's Vegetable Recipes

Spinach & Artichoke Stuffed Tomato

1 ¾ cups canned artichoke hearts (canned in
    spring water)
½ lb. spinach fresh or frozen
2 teaspoons of fat-free butter spray or
    Benecol® Spread
8–10 fresh basil leaves, roughly chopped.
½ cup chicken broth
½–1 teaspoon black pepper
½–1 teaspoon salt
½–1 teaspoon garlic powder
3–4 medium-sized tomatoes, cored, with
    seeds and pulp removed

To core tomato: Angle a sharp knife at a 45 degree angle and cut towards the center about ¾ of the length of the tomato to shape an inverted cone.

In a sauté pan, simmer the artichoke hearts in chicken broth for 5–8 minutes until tender. Add garlic powder, salt , black pepper, Benecol® Spread or butter spray. Cook for 5–8 minutes. Fill prepared tomatoes. Season and finish with basil. Chill and serve cold or bake at 375 degrees for 10 minutes to serve it hot.

Onion Squash

8–9 yellow or summer squash
½ onion, roughly chopped
¼ cup chicken broth
2 tablespoons fat-free butter spray or
    Benecol® Spread
1 teaspoon salt
1 teaspoon black pepper

Lightly coat a sauté pan with non-stick cooking spray (the pan must have a cover). Heat to med-high. Cook the onions 3–5 minutes until they begin to brown. Add ¼ cup of chicken broth and the squash. Cover and cook for 5–8 minutes. Season with salt and black pepper. Serve.

LEMON BROCCOLI

1–2 broccoli crowns
1 lemon
1 tablespoon Benecol® spread or
    Fat-free Butter Spray
1 teaspoon Cajun/Creole seasoning mix or
    black pepper
1 teaspoon salt

Cut broccoli into pieces that are a little larger than "bite sized." Place the cut broccoli in a covered microwavable dish with 2–3 tablespoons of water. Microwave for four minutes. Let the broccoli stand while covered for 1–2 minutes. Pour out the water. Add the remaining ingredients and toss the broccoli. Sprinkle lemon juice over the top. Serve.

CRISPY FRESH GREEN BEANS

4 cups fresh green beans (snap or cut ends
    off before cooking)
Non-stick cooking spray
1 tablespoon Benecol® Spread or fat-free
    butter spray
1 teaspoon Cajun/Creole seasoning mix or
    black pepper
1 teaspoon salt
Lemon juice
1 large bowl of chilled water with ice

Lightly coat a large saucepan or pot with non-stick cooking spray. Heat to med-high. Saute the green beans in the pan until the color changes to a light green. Remove the green beans immediately and place into the bowl of cold water to stop the cooking process. Strain the green beans. Heat the same pan and add the green beans back with all the remaining ingredients until the green beans are warm. Immediately remove from heat and serve.

SALAD DRESSINGS

HOT MUSTARD SALAD

¼ onion
½ bell pepper
1 cup chicken broth
2 tablespoons mustard powder (may substitute Dijon or Creole mustard)
1 tablespoon balsamic or red wine vinegar
1 tablespoon cracked or Malabar black pepper
2 teaspoons salt
Romaine lettuce

Lightly spray pan with non-stick butter flavor cooking spray.

On med-high heat, sauté the onions and bell peppers until browning begins. Add broth and cook down until the liquid becomes thick. Remove from the heat. Add mustard and all remaining ingredients except the romaine lettuce. Once mixed, pour the dressing over romaine lettuce and toss. Serve with hot dressing or chill the dressing prior to tossing for a cold salad.

LOW-CALORIE HERB VINAIGRETTE

3 tablespoons Creole mustard
¼ cup balsamic vinegar
½ teaspoon thyme (dried)
½ teaspoon basil (dried)
1 teaspoon cracked black pepper or Malabar black pepper
¼ cup chopped green onions
¼ cup parsley
½ teaspoon salt

Mix all ingredients together until consistent. Drizzle over romaine or your favorite mixed greens.

RASPBERRY VINAIGRETTE

¼ cup fresh raspberries
3 tablespoons Creole mustard
¼ cup balsamic vinegar
½ teaspoon thyme (dried)
½ teaspoon basil (dried)
1 teaspoon cracked black pepper or Malabar
    black pepper
¼ cup chopped green onions
¼ cup parsley
½ teaspoon salt

Puree raspberries in a blender. Strain puree to remove seeds. Add all remaining ingredients. Blend & drizzle over romaine lettuce or your favorite mixed greens.

MARY — GETTING KIDS TO EAT VEGETABLES

Mary is a loving mother whose kids sneer at vegetables and scream for pizza. Knowing the long-term health problems associated with poor nutrition, Mary developed a plan to change their eating habits.

First, she made the kids a deal that they could eat pizza twice a week if they had a PrescriptFit™ shake or pudding before and if they added one vegetable choice for every meat choice on their pizza.

Eventually she convinced the family to make pizza together, a fun activity that offered the bonus of making Mary more of a "culinary expert" in the household.

Two years later, Mary's kids are eating five cups of vegetables daily and paying a lot more attention to Mom's ideas on calories, nutrition, cooking, and what tastes "good."

Mary exhibited the patience and understanding necessary to change her family's eating habits. Habits and preferences are developed with practice. They take time, but are worth it!

CASE STUDY

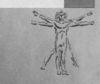

~ Section B: Diving In... ~

Reminder:

- Continue 6–8 or more PrescriptFit™ amino acid doses per day.
- Use PrescriptFit™ shakes or soups before or with meals.
- Use foods from Phases 2–5.
- Take a multi-vitamin supplement.
- Drink 5 cups of water or calorie-free beverage daily.

PHASE 5 EGGS

By now, if you've been following the PrescriptFit™ MNT Plan, you are probably eager for each new Food Phase, for it adds to the variety of foods from which you can plan your meals.

EGGS AND NUTRITION

Eggs are a wonderful addition to your meal planning for they are low in calories, filling, provide added taste and texture, and may be mixed with Food Phase 1–4 foods to create new recipes. Eggs do not cause dangerous insulin resistance or blood vessel malfunction. Eggs are high in protein and relatively low in fat, especially if the yolk is removed. However, egg yolk does contain a number of essential vitamins, and it is not necessary to always remove the yolk. Eggs are very inexpensive and can meet any budget. Eggs are for unlimited consumption. All you can eat!

EGG MYTHS

The most stubborn myth about eggs is the concern that high cholesterol levels found in egg yolk will lead to atherosclerosis (cholesterol artery plaque). While the yolk does contain high amounts of cholesterol,

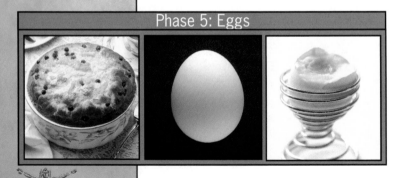

Phase 5: Eggs

The Amino Solution
©2009 Stanford A. Owen, MD

cholesterol in food does not result in elevated blood cholesterol levels. Rather, sugar and saturated fat are the culprits that provoke the liver to manufacture and over-produce cholesterol. Dietary cholesterol alone, when consumed without saturated fat or sugar, may actually decrease cholesterol production by the liver. For those skeptical about egg safety, simply limit egg consumption to three or fewer eggs per week.

Dosing:
No restriction — Enjoy eggs alone, in omelets with vegetables, or in mixed dishes based on what phase of the Plan you are currently following.

The true calorie danger in egg dishes comes with the addition of condiments. Avoid using cheese when preparing egg dishes. Cheese is composed mostly of saturated fat and is high calorie.

CALORIES AND EGGS

Calories range between 80 and 90 calories per egg. For ease of remembering, just round it off to 100. One egg equals 100 calories, which would require one mile of walking for "payback."

Egg yolk contains fat (at 9 calories/gram of fat). Egg white is pure protein (at 4 calories/gram). To cut back on calories, remove the yolk.

PrescriptFit Egg Pro™ product is pure egg-white powder. Egg Pro™ can be mixed with PrescriptFit™ shakes and soups or omelets to give more body and satiation. Egg white contains large amounts of the branched-chain amino acids that improve metabolism.

☙ *Section B: Diving In...* ☙

BOB OWEN'S EGG RECIPES

HARD BOILED EGGS

Place eggs in pan and add enough cold water to cover by 1 inch. Cover and quickly bring to a boil. Reduce heat to a simmer and cook for 5 minutes.

Rinse in cold water, let stand for 5 minutes. Then, rinse again in cold water, let stand or place in refrigerator.

SOFT BOILED EGGS

Place eggs in pan and add enough water to cover by 1 inch. Remove eggs and bring water to a boil.

With slotted spoon, place eggs in water, and continue to cook for 3–4 minutes. Immediately remove eggs with a slotted spoon and rinse with cold water.

Place eggs for 1 minute or less in ice water. Carefully test the heat. If too hot to handle, place in ice water again.

With a knife, lightly crack the egg and carefully peel. Slice the egg as you desire.

POACHED EGGS

In a small saucepan, bring 2 inches water to a boil; add 1 teaspoon vinegar. Reduce to a gentle simmer. Break an egg into a saucer. Holding the saucer just above simmering water, gently slip egg into saucepan. Continue for remaining eggs. Cook in barely simmering water 3 to 5 minutes.

Remove the eggs with a slotted spoon; trim the edges if needed. Set on warm plates.

Deviled Eggs

6 eggs
1 ½ tablespoons mustard (Creole or
   French's® Grey Poupon
1 tablespoon lemon juice
1 tablespoon pickle relish or finely chopped
   jalapenos
1 tablespoon Worcestershire sauce
1 tablespoon finely chopped green onions
   or chives
⅛ teaspoon salt
¼ teaspoon black pepper or Cajun/Creole
   seasoning mix
¼ teaspoon paprika

Hard boil the eggs and let them cool. Cut the
eggs into two halves long ways. Separate the
yolks into a small mixing bowl and place the
egg whites on a tray. Combine the mustard,
lemon juice, Worcestershire sauce, green
onions, salt, pepper, and paprika with the eggs
yolks and mix thoroughly. Spoon the mixture
into the egg whites and sprinkle with a little
paprika. Chill for about half an hour and serve.

Mushroom Omelet with Rosemary

2 cups sliced fresh mushrooms
2 eggs
1 tablespoon minced rosemary
Black pepper (a dash)
Salt (a dash)
1 ½ – 2 tablespoons green onions finely
   chopped
1 tablespoon fresh parsley—finely chopped
Non-stick butter flavor cooking spray

In a small bowl, beat together 2 eggs and
seasoning until blended. Coat a 7- to 10-inch
non-stick omelet pan with non-stick butter
flavored cooking spray. Heat on med-high
until just hot enough to sizzle a drop of

water. Saute mushrooms, rosemary, and green onions until cooked.

Pour in egg mixture. (Mixture should set immediately at edges.) When top begins to thicken, gently loosen the omelet around the edges. Flip one side over the other with a spatula. Flip the omelet to cook on opposite side.

Invert the pan to drop the omelet onto the plate with a quick flip of the wrist or slide from pan onto plate. Season with salt & pepper. Sprinkle with green onions and parsley.

PEPPERED PICKLED EGGS

    8 hard-cooked eggs, peeled
    1 ½ cups white vinegar
    ¼ cup water
    4–5 whole peppers – cayenne, jalapeno,
        habanera, or personal preference
    1 teaspoon black peppercorns
    1 teaspoon salt

Arrange eggs in 1-quart jar with tight-fitting lid. In medium saucepan, stir together all remaining ingredients. Bring to boiling. Reduce heat and gently simmer 5 minutes.

Pour hot mixture over eggs. Cover tightly. Store in cool place OR cool at room temperature for 1 hour. Refrigerate to blend flavors, at least several days or up to several weeks. After opening, refrigerate and use within 1 week.

EGGATELLA FLORENTINE

    3 ½ cups canned chicken broth
    1 package (10 oz.) frozen chopped spinach
    1 teaspoon salt
    Black pepper
    Thyme
    1 bay leaf

Paul Prudhomme's Magic Seasoning Blend®
1 teaspoon fat-free butter spray or Benecol®
4 eggs, well beaten
¼ cup grated Parmesan cheese
1 tablespoon finely chopped green onions
1 teaspoon chopped garlic

In a large saucepan over high heat, bring broth to a boil. Add spinach. Cook until thawed, stirring occasionally with fork to separate. Stir in seasoning, butter spray, and garlic. Reduce heat to simmering. While stirring soup, slowly pour in eggs. Immediately remove from heat. Pour or ladle about 1 cup soup into each of six (10-ounce) bowls. Sprinkle each with 1 tablespoon of the cheese and green onions.

Harold — A New Twist on the "Farm-Style" Breakfast

Harold came to our clinic to lose weight after suffering a heart attack. His cholesterol level was high; yet, he was essentially unaware of what cholesterol truly is and what can be done to control it. The only thing he was certain of was that cholesterol played a role in his heart attack, that the dietician at the hospital told him to avoid eggs, and that this was going to be a difficult change to make.

Having to give up the kind of breakfast he'd always known — sausage, eggs, biscuits, juice, whole milk — was very distressing for Harold. Moreover, his breakfast was a special time for him: a time of day spent with his wife (while the kids were still asleep).

I explained to Harold how current science has shown that the cytokine-provoking saturated fat in the sausage, biscuit, and whole milk was inflamed even further by the simple sugar in the biscuit and juice. It wasn't really the eggs that were the culprits in his "farm-style" breakfast; in fact, the cholesterol-like molecules in egg yolk might even be working to "turn off" cholesterol production by the liver.

Harold's wife came up with some creative substitutes — turkey sausage and a PrescriptFit™ shake for the pork sausage and whole milk and sugar-free Crystal Light™ instead of juice. She also eliminated the biscuit. Harold focused on cooking omelets and other egg dishes and became quite the chef. His cholesterol and weight dropped to normal ranges within six months without feeling deprived.

CASE STUDY

Section B: Diving In...

PHASE 6 NUTS

You may eat any variety of nuts on the PrescriptFit™ MNT Plan. All varieties are available year-round and each has its own unique flavor and texture. You can buy most nuts either shelled or unshelled. Unshelled nuts make great snacks, especially for the kids. Shell-cracking takes time (which limits caloric intake) and can be fun (or at least mesmerizing). Unshelled nuts may cost a little less.

Nuts are often considered snacks or party food, but they are especially useful as condiments on meat, vegetables, and dessert dishes.

NUTS AS NUTRITION

You may wonder why nuts, which are higher in fat, are added ahead of fruit in the Food Phase plan. There are several reasons:

- Nuts contain no carbohydrates and will not cause insulin resistance.
- Nut oils improve small blood vessel function, aiding in blood pressure and circulation.
- The thin covering of certain nuts contain substances that lower cholesterol overall

Categories of Nuts

Walnuts, pecans, almonds, pistachio, peanuts, cashews, pine nuts, hickory nuts, chestnuts, acorns, Brazil nuts, hazelnuts

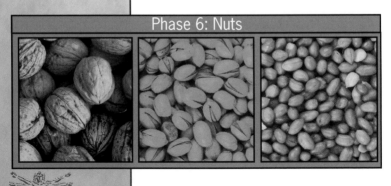

Phase 6: Nuts

Dosing:
Nuts are one of the highest calorie/ounce foods at an average 175 calories per ounce. However, studies have demonstrated no weight gain in lean or obese individuals using nuts without restriction as a daily snack for six months. If you are susceptible to binge eating, you'll want to be extra careful with nuts. You should use primarily unshelled nuts or limit shelled nuts to no more than ¼ cup per day.

by raising "good" HDL cholesterol and lowering "bad" LDL cholesterol.

- While nuts are rich in oil (oil is 125 calories/tablespoon), one third of nut oil is not absorbed, instead passing through the intestine bound to nut fiber.

- Nuts are very satiating because nuts are high in protein and fat.

NUT MYTHS

Salted nuts contain no more calories than unsalted nuts. However, you may need to avoid salted nuts if you have a medical condition that involves sensitivity to salt, such as congestive heart failure, kidney failure, and hypertension.

In addition to shelled or unshelled, salted or unsalted, you can also buy some nuts ground to use as a spread. Beware, however, that commercial peanut butter is often mixed with hydrogenated vegetable oil ("trans fat") to enhance texture, which ruins the health benefits of the nuts. If you have a health food store nearby, see if they have nut grinders for fresh nut spread.

⊱ Section B: Diving In... ⊰

BOB OWEN'S NUT RECIPES

TOASTED ALMONDS

1 cup cracked or sliced almonds
Non-stick cooking spray
Table salt

Lightly coat a baking sheet with non-stick cooking spray. Lay almonds flat on the sheet, and place in the oven. Broil for 2-3 minutes or until the whites of the almonds begin to turn light brown. Turn the almonds over and repeat the process on the uncooked side, taking care not to burn the almonds. Remove from oven, and sprinkle with salt.

CANDIED PECANS

2–4 cups of pecans
2 packets of Splenda®
1 tablespoon of Benecol® spread
1 teaspoon each of vanilla & brandy extract
1 teaspoon of cinnamon
2–3 dashes of nutmeg
1 dash salt
½ cup water

In a saucepan or small pot, combine ingredients except pecans. Heat until mixture dissolves; add pecans and stir until covered. Remove from heat; lay flat on wax paper/baking sheet to cool. Serve.

SALTED WALNUTS

2–4 cups walnut pieces
3 tablespoons salt
1 teaspoon sugar
2 tablespoons Benecol® spread

In a small pot or saucepan, add butter, salt and sugar. Heat on medium until dissolved. Remove the pot from the heat. Add the walnuts and stir until covered. Lay the walnuts flat on wax paper or a baking sheet until cool. Serve.

Phase 7 Fruit

Some of you who love fruit are now saying, "Ah, at last I can add fruit to my meal plan!" Others of you may have learned to fear fruit for its carbohydrate content. Fruit should not be feared, but it is added in the second half of the PrescriptFit™ MNT Plan since fruit is primarily carbohydrate. If you have a medical condition sensitive to sugar, you'll want to ask your health care provider to monitor your condition closely during Food Phase 7.

Fruit as Nutrition

Fresh fruit contains carbohydrate and fiber as primary nutrients. Some fruits contain small amounts of fat (avocado). Fruits also contain vitamins and minerals, especially vitamin C, and minimal amounts of protein.

Although you can get the same amount of vitamins and minerals in pills with zero calories, and the same amount of fiber from food supplement powders, natural fruit has its advantages. For one thing, it has "entertainment" value because it tastes good. Unlike other entertainment foods that contain processed sugars, the sugar in fruit is contained and intertwined with the fiber, causing a slow release of the sugar into the

Reminder:

- Continue 6–8 or more PrescriptFit™ amino acid doses per day.
- Use PrescriptFit™ shakes or soups before or with meals.
- Use foods from Phases 2–7.
- Take a multi-vitamin supplement.
- Drink 5 cups of water or calorie-free beverage daily.

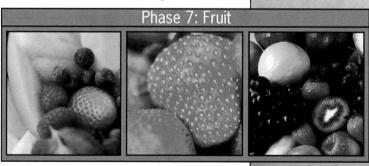

Phase 7: Fruit

The Amino Solution
©2009 Stanford A. Owen, MD

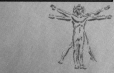

Dosing:
If fruit is raw or whole, "overdose" on fruit calories is very unlikely. Therefore, the PrescriptFit™ MNT Plan does not restrict fruit consumption.

bloodstream — a phenomenon known as "glycemic index." The more rapidly sugar enters the bloodstream after a meal, the higher the glycemic index.

All fruit has a relatively low glycemic index compared to "high glycemic index" soft drinks, juices, and snacks. Fruit can satisfy your "sweet tooth" without the huge doses of sugar from refined products. How many pieces of fruit would it take to squeeze one glass of orange, grapefruit, grape, pineapple, apple, or other juices? Imagine eating that many pieces of fruit in the 30 seconds it takes you to gulp down a glass of juice or soda! If you replace one refined snack or glass of juice with piece of fresh fruit, the benefit is huge.

CATEGORIES OF FRUIT

There are too many categories or varieties of fruit to name here. Challenge yourself and your family to try new fruits along with the familiar and customary varieties you may already eat regularly. If you are already accustomed to eating oranges, apples, bananas, grapes, strawberries, or melon, try kiwi or blueberries. Remember to experiment with a variety of colors. As you try new varieties of fruit, ask each member of the family for their opinion. Kids, in particular, are open to new tastes if challenged with variety early in life. Don't make a big deal about the "new" fruit. Instead be a role model for your family, willing to try new tastes, and express your reaction with adjectives like "yummy" or "phenomenal."

CALORIES IN FRUIT

Fruit calories are measured in ounces, from 5 calories per ounce (lemon and tomato) to 45 calories per ounce (avocado). These are very low calories per ounce compared to almost any other food choice. Even avocado, at 45 calories per ounce, is less than chicken (50 calories per ounce). The reason fruit is placed in Food Phase 7, rather than an earlier Food Phase, is that fruit is not very satiating. Fruit does not "fill" or "stick to the ribs," so eating fruit will not usually reduce overall calorie intake; you'll still feel hungry for something else. Fruit is very tasty and should be considered a "treat" for the sweet tooth.

Thousands of fruit varieties from all parts of the world are now available in our local stores. If a particular fruit is not listed below, guess which type it would be most similar to.

Fruit is low in calories per ounce. Use the chart below to compare the caloric content of your favorite fruits. If a particular fruit is not listed, ask yourself if it is more like one of those listed below.

FRUIT	CALORIES/OUNCE	AMOUNT = TO ABOUT 100 CALORIES OR BURNED IN WALKING ONE MILE
Lemon, Tomato	5	20 ounces
Melons	10	¼ watermelon
Apple, Pineapple, Orange	15	2
Grapes	20	One large bowl
Banana	30	One banana
Avocado	45	About ½ avocado
Dried fruit	85	Avoid as is very calorie-dense when limiting calories

Section B: Diving In...

It is more important to enjoy a particular fruit than "sweat" the calories. If you and your family enjoy a fruit, you are more likely to consume them daily and forego less nutritious snacks.

Keep fruit in front of your face from Food Phase 7 forward. Replace refined sugar snacks with fruit, nuts, or PrescriptFit™ snack bars. Place them on the counter, in the den, and around the television or computer.

Buy and mix as many colors and varieties as possible. Each color represents different nutrients and vitamins, different tastes, and additional options for the picky eaters in your family.

BOB OWEN'S FRUIT RECIPES

BAKED PEARS

THE GROCERY LIST

- Pears
- Apples
- Vanilla extract
- Lemon juice
- Pineapple
- Tangerine or Mandarin oranges
- Tea or coffee — Mix sugar substitute, PrescriptFit™ vanilla flavor, and a bit of water for coffee creamer

2–4 peeled, cored cooking pears, cut in half
2 packets Splenda®
1 tablespoon Benecol® Spread or fat free
    butter spray
1 teaspoon cinnamon
1 teaspoon vanilla extract
2–3 dashes of nutmeg
1 teaspoon lemon juice
2–3 dashes of salt
2 cups water

Preheat oven to 375 degrees. In a baking dish, mix all ingredients except pears until combined. Add pears to pan. Bake in the oven for 35 minutes, basting pears every 7–10 minutes. Remove from oven, baste with sauce, and serve.

Sweet Apples

> 3–5 cored, sliced apples (Granny Smith,
>   Macintosh, Fuji recommended)
> Non-stick cooking spray
> 2 packets Splenda®
> 2 tablespoons of fat free butter spray or
>   Benecol® spread
> 1 teaspoon cinnamon
> 1 teaspoon vanilla extract
> 2–3 dashes of salt
> 2–3 dashes of nutmeg
> 1 teaspoon lemon juice

Lightly coat a saucepan or small pot with non-stick cooking spray. Heat pan to medium. Add the apples and cook for 2–3 minutes or until the apples begin to soften. Add the remaining ingredients and cook for an additional 3 minutes or until the apples begin to fall apart. Serve hot or refrigerate and serve cold.

Citrus Mix

> 2–3 Satsuma, tangerine, or mandarin
>   oranges, peeled and pulled into pieces
> 1 lemon, peeled and quartered
> ½ pineapple, cut into slices
> 2 packets Splenda®
> ½ cup water

In a saucepan, combine the water and Splenda®. Heat on medium until simmering. Add the fruit and toss for 1–2 minutes until slightly warm. Serve.

The Amino Solution
©2009 Stanford A. Owen, MD

*Section B: Diving In... *

Reminder:

- Continue 6–8 or more PrescriptFit™ amino acid doses per day.
- Use PrescriptFit™ shakes or soups before or with meals.
- Use foods from Phases 2–8.
- Take a multi-vitamin supplement.
- Drink 5 cups of water or calorie-free beverage daily.

PHASE 8: PRESCRIPTFIT™ SNACKS

Snacks are a part of modern Western culture. For some people snacks are so handy and tempting they lead to unconscious over-consumption. The solution is usually not to deprive ourselves of snacks but to learn to choose snacks that are healthy alternatives.

All PrescriptFit™ snacks are high in protein, low in glycemic sugars (sucrose), and they taste good! You'll probably find that you can replace your typical household snacks for kids and spouses with PrescriptFit™ snack bars. If you're doubtful, don't tell them that you are using "diet food," and see if they notice the difference. More than likely, they'll demand you keep these items around, making your diet tasks easier.

In addition to PrescriptFit™ snacks, you can always use fruits and nuts as healthy snack alternatives.

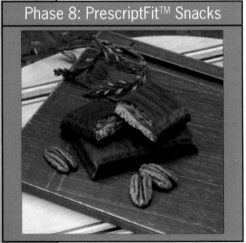

Phase 8: PrescriptFit™ Snacks

The Amino Solution
©2009 Stanford A. Owen, MD

Most PrescriptFit™ snacks are made from nonfat dry milk, egg white, soy proteins, and artificial sweeteners. The chocolate snack is made from the highest quality cocoa, an excellent antioxidant that has direct beneficial effects on small blood vessels. You may also use these products as a dessert or as a meal replacement. A shake and snack bar is a filling meal. Unless consumed in large quantities, snack bars should not induce cytokine production from fat cells.

PrescriptFit™ bars taste as good as candy bars, but they are far different. Commercial candy bars are made with sucrose (sugar) and large amounts of hydrogenated vegetable oils. They are huge, with 3–4 times the calories as PrescriptFit™ snack bars.

If chips and pastries are your weakness, consider this: All varieties have about 125 calories per ounce. And if you are one who "can't eat just one," those calories will add up quickly, along with the fat. You'll be much more successful at achieving and maintaining your desired weight and fitness level if you ban the chips and pastries and choose fruit, nuts, or PrescriptFit™ bars instead.

Dosing:
Unlimited. For an extra treat, crumble a PrescriptFit™ bar over a PrescriptFit™ pudding.

PRESCRIPTFIT™ SNACK BARS

All PrescriptFit™ Snack Bars average about 150 calories. All are high protein (about 50 percent), very satiating, and they taste great.

The bars can be used as a snack or meal replacement. Protein content is soy, egg white, and milk solids. A snack bar and shake is great choice for lunch, after school snack, or for dessert!

Try these bar flavors:

- Crisp N' Crunch Cinnamon
- Crisp N' Crunch Peanut Bar
- Crisp N' Crunch Double Berry
- Crisp N' Crunch Fudge Graham
- Crisp N' Crunch Cocoa Café
- Coconut
- Toffee
- Chocolate Mint
- Lemon Crunch
- Butter Pecan
- Brownie
- Chocolate Chip Cookie Dough
- Cookies and Cream
- Double Chocolate
- Oatmeal Cinnamon Raisin

The Amino Solution
©2009 Stanford A. Owen, MD

Section B: Diving In...

CASE STUDY

Splurging and The Amino Solution

The "splurge" meal concept was developed after polling patients in our clinic about how many high-calorie, high-fat, "fun" (as described by those polled) meals are absolutely essential for quality life. From this poll, we reached two, overwhelming conclusions:

1. Ninety percent of those polled stated that five to ten meals per month were "essential." Their comments frequently sounded like this, "I live in the New Orleans area, where food is a crucial ingredient of our way of life. It is as essential as the music to our festivities and culture as a whole."

   In New Orleans, eating is entertainment. Yet, most New Orleanians agree that two to three meals per week at a world-class eatery is adequate (even if price is not an issue). Give this some thought, and ask your spouse or friends. Most will agree.

2. Participants who recorded splurge meals for the coming month had something of an "epiphany." When actually writing down all the unexpected but planned events that resulted in "splurging," people could easily see what accounted for the many pounds gained in a given year.

All participants of the poll used the PrescriptFit™ Calendar. If you can't seem to determine where those extra pounds came from, use the PrescriptFit™ Calendar — it works!

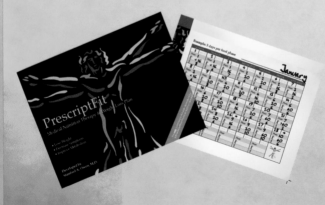

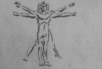

CHAPTER 7: LET'S SPLURGE! — PHASES 9–13

SPECIAL MEALS FOR SPECIAL OCCASIONS

Merriam-Webster Dictionary defines the verb, "to splurge" as "To indulge oneself extravagantly." Whether we are being extravagant with our money, say, indulging in a new outfit, or extravagant with our food choices, it is not something we do every day. If we did, we wouldn't get that special thrill we feel when we break through our normal restraints and behave extravagantly!

In the context of the Amino Solution, we use "splurging" to describe a special meal, usually involving entertainment or social interaction. Generally, most meals used for such purposes are higher in fat, carbohydrate, and calories than the routine meals that have become our norm on the Food Phase Plan.

Most restaurant meals would be considered "splurge" meals. Most family feasts are splurge meals. Some business meetings might qualify as splurge meals. Many vacation meals would be splurge meals. Life crises definitely throw unplanned meals your way. I call "splurge" meals my "Weekends, Weddings, and Wakes" solution.

Alcoholic beverages are also considered "splurge" items. Alcohol is usually consumed in high-calorie environments and will lower inhibitions in anyone attempting food

Medical Treatment

The Amino Solution

Splurging

Healing & Education

> *Eight splurge meals are allowed every month.*

avoidance — so why try? Go with it. Add the alcohol to the "splurge" and pay back later.

"Splurge" meals should be enjoyed. Do not restrict portions. Do not strain your brain. Try to plan "splurge" meals through the month by placing them on your PrescriptFit™ Calendar at the beginning of the month. BUT if a "splurge" opportunity comes your way unplanned, enjoy the event. Simply replace a previously planned "splurge" meal on the Calendar the following day. For many, this will be an eye-opening experience. It may take practice and patience to hold total "splurge" meals to eight or less per month.

Splurging also allows for extended diet distractions, such as a vacation or life crisis. All eight splurge meals may be used consecutively for an extended trip or vacation. When, not if, a crisis hits, the splurge meals can also be counted consecutively until you're through the crisis. Simply replace future splurge meals until they are balanced out. This may take several months. No big deal!

Splurging is a unique concept of the Plan. The simple fact is eight meals per month out of a potential ninety meal slots (3 meals per day times 30 days per month) is not going to make someone obese or drastically alter their disease stability.

Splurging allows you to integrate your real life with your structured diet plan. It works!

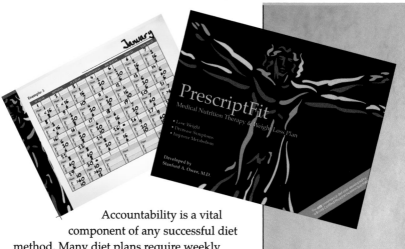

Accountability is a vital component of any successful diet method. Many diet plans require weekly meetings to enforce accountability. With the Amino Solution, you hold yourself accountable by using the PrescriptFit™ Calendar. (See pages 36–37 for complete directions on using the Calendar.)

Mark your anticipated "splurge" meals on your Calendar at the beginning of the month. When you have unanticipated splurging, mark those meals on the calendar and remove a planned splurge meal. If you update your Calendar daily, you will be accountable daily, not weekly, for your success or failure. Demonstrate accountability to your physician by bringing your disease/symptom questionnaires (from section C) to your physician appointments.

Role model accountability for your family and friends by sharing your strategies and results. You never know how you might help others improve their own health by being a positive example.

If real people are going to follow a diet plan forever, the diet plan has to function in the real world. Splurging and feasting are as old as civilization. Our entire culture is built around feasting, family, and friends. Any diet that does not consider this fact will fail.

Section B: Diving In...

Reminder:

- Continue 6–8 or more PrescriptFit™ amino acid doses per day.
- Use PrescriptFit™ shakes or soups before or with meals.
- Use foods from Phases 2–8.
- Use Phase 9 food for splurges ONLY.
- Take a multi-vitamin supplement.
- Drink 5 cups of water or calorie-free beverage daily.

PHASE 9 PORK

Promoters call pork, "the other white meat," referring to poultry or fish. However, pork is not poultry or fish. Even the leanest cuts of pork have substantial saturated fat and calories. Pork is pork and should not be substituted for poultry or fish as a major component of your diet.

PORK AS NUTRITION

Pork and beef could be considered nutritionally comparable. They are placed in separate Food Phases primarily to encourage skill training with recipes. Pork varies in fat content with cut and individual carcass fat. Pork from wild hogs is quite lean, approaching fat content in poultry. Commercially raised pork averages 100–125 calories per ounce.

Pork contains no carbohydrate. The leanest port cut (pork loin) averages about 100 calories/ounce. You can trim some of the calories by trimming away any visible excess fat. However, most fat is mingled or "marbleized" into pork meat and cannot be easily removed with trimming.

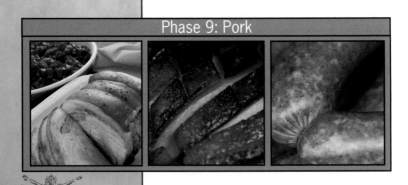

Phase 9: Pork

Pork fat is saturated fat that
induces the liver to
manufacture excessive
cholesterol, especially
the "bad" or harmful
LDL cholesterol
particles that inflame
arteries. Saturated fat
induces insulin malfunction or
"resistance," increases cytokine production, and
impairs small blood vessel function, leading to
hypertension and fluid retention.

Dosing — Splurge Only!
Because pork is high in calories and
harmful saturated fat, it should be consumed
at "splurge" meals, no more than eight
per month.

Some individuals are more sensitive to the
adverse effects of saturated fat than others.
Those with heart attack or stroke in the family,
elevated cholesterol levels, diabetes, or pre-
diabetes (IRS), should be especially careful when
adding the pork Food Phase to the Plan. If you
have diabetes, pre-diabetes, or heart disease,
work with your health care provider to monitor
blood pressure, sudden increase in scale weight
(fluid retention), blood sugar, cholesterol, and
triglycerides.

CATEGORIES OF PORK AND CALORIES

Pork is made from hogs; preparation of the
meat results in different fat or calorie content.

- Ham (smoked pork treated with sugar)
- Sausage (ground pork, usually with
  added fat)
- Deli meats (processed pork)
- Chops and roasts

Pork averages between 100 and 125 calories
per ounce, with pork loin on the lean end and
pork chops on the fatter end of pork cuts.
Sausage tops out at about 150 calories/ounce
(about the same as heavy pies or cheesecake).

☞ *Section B: Diving In...* ☜

Cooking Tip:
Pork mixes well with chicken, shrimp, and vegetables. Amino Solution recipes merge the flavor of pork with other foods to gain the flavor but not too many calories and saturated fat.

SPLURGING WITH PORK

Mark your PrescriptFit™ Calendar at the beginning of each month and mark off eight allowed "splurge" meals. Plan a splurge meal with pork where you can:

- Eat as much of the splurge item(s) as desired but only for that meal.

- Mix pork with foods from Food Phases 1–8 to achieve calorie balance and to limit "damage" from that splurge meal.

BOB OWEN'S PORK RECIPES

SMOTHERED PORK TENDERLOIN

1 pork tenderloin, sliced in round steaks
1 onion, chopped
1 green bell pepper, chopped
1 Knorr® bouillon cube,
    dissolved in 1 cup water
1 bay leaf
¼ cup PrescriptFit™ Chicken Soup mixed in
    ¼ cup of water
Non-stick cooking spray
Cajun / Creole seasoning mix or black
    pepper
Salt

Dust the pork steaks with seasonings. Lightly coat a large sauté pan with non-stick cooking spray and heat to medium-high. Brown the pork steaks on both sides. Remove pork and set aside. Add the onions and bell peppers to the same pan, and sauté all ingredients for 1–2 minutes. Return the pork to the same pan. Add the bay leaf and the dissolved bouillon. Cover and cook for 15–20 minutes or until the bell peppers mute in color. Add the PrescriptFit™ Chicken soup to the sauce, and mix until a gravy forms. Serve.

ASIAN PORK

1 lb. pork tenderloin, fat trimmed from meat
¼ cup low-sodium soy sauce
1 teaspoon cinnamon
2 tablespoons rice wine vinegar
3 green onions, chopped
2 cloves garlic, minced
1 teaspoon Splenda®
1 tablespoon grated fresh ginger (see
Cooking Tip, at right)

Cooking Tip:

When you buy fresh ginger, select smooth, firm, unblemished roots. Slice off just what you need from the root. Peel away the brown outer layer, and working against the grain, chop, grate, or slice the fibrous flesh.

Whisk together soy sauce and remaining ingredients in a small bowl; pour over steak. Marinate in the refrigerator 1 hour, turning occasionally. Broil the tenderloin on the oven rack using a broiler pan. The tenderloin should sit in the center of the rack at least 5 inches from the burners. Cook 5 minutes or more on each side or to your satisfaction. Let stand 5 minutes. To cut: Slice across the grain in a downward, diagonal motion.

BARBECUED PORK LOIN

1 pork tenderloin
2 tablespoons barbecue sauce
2 teaspoons paprika
2 teaspoons salt
½ teaspoon pepper
½ teaspoon garlic powder
1 teaspoon onion powder
1 tablespoon Worcestershire sauce
½ teaspoon Tabasco® or other hot pepper
sauce
½ cup lemon juice (3 to 4 lemons)
1 cup vinegar
1 cup water

Place pork loin roast in a roasting pan. In a medium saucepan, combine paprika, salt, pepper, garlic powder, onion powder, Worcestershire sauce, pepper sauce, lemon juice, vinegar, and water; bring to boiling

⤳ *Section B: Diving In...* ⤳

point. Spoon some sauce over meat. Roast pork loin at 325° for about 2 to 2 ½ hours, or to an internal temperature of at least 160° on a meat thermometer. Baste pork frequently with the sauce.

Rosemary Roasted Pork Tenderloin

> 1 pork tenderloin (about 1 pound)
> 3 tablespoons minced fresh rosemary, or
>   about 1 tablespoon dried
> 2 cloves garlic, halved
> Salt and pepper to taste
> Non-stick cooking spray

Preheat oven to 400°. Line a baking pan with foil, spray with cooking spray and place in oven. Trim fat from pork tenderloins and butterfly the meat, cutting them nearly in half lengthwise. Open the pork tenderloins and lay out, pounding to flatten with the palm of the hand or the bottom of a heavy skillet. Chop rosemary if using fresh.

Rub pork tenderloins all over with cut sides of garlic halves, and then sprinkle rosemary on both sides. Remove baking pan from the oven and place pork on hot tray. Return to oven and roast for about 20 minutes (about 155–160° internal temp). Remove and let stand five minutes, then slice.

The Amino Solution
©2009 Stanford A. Owen, MD

PHASE 10 BEEF

Beef is easily America's favorite food. But because beef is loaded with harmful saturated fat and calories, and is easily consumed to excess, consider it a "splurge" item for your monthly food calendar.

> *Dosing — Splurge Only!*
> *Because beef is high in calories and harmful saturated fat, it should be consumed at "splurge" meals, no more than eight per month.*

BEEF AS NUTRITION

Beef contains no carbohydrates and is composed mainly of protein and fat. The fat is "marbleized" into the meat. If you "fry" beef, little extra fat enters the meat since it is already saturated. To minimize calories, trim excess fat from the meat prior to cooking.

Lean cuts of beef (round roasts or steak, chuck) have approximately 100 calories per ounce while heavier cuts of beef (sirloin, rib-eye, T-bone) average about 125 calories per ounce. Cooking the fat out of the meat is helpful to reduce the calories, but why bother? If you are going to use beef as a "treat" (eight splurge meals per month), why remove the substance that provides the "treat" — the fat?

Reminder:
- Continue 6–8 or more PrescriptFit™ amino acid doses per day.
- Use PrescriptFit™ shakes or soups before or with meals.
- Use foods from Phases 2–8.
- Use Phase 10 food for splurges ONLY.
- Take a multi-vitamin supplement.
- Drink 5 cups of water or calorie-free beverage daily.

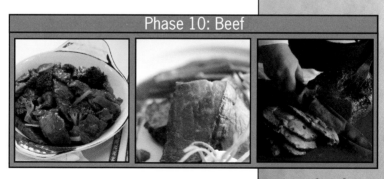

Phase 10: Beef

The Amino Solution
©2009 Stanford A. Owen, MD

☞ Section B: Diving In... ☜

Combine beef with other foods for healthier splurge meals. "Medley" recipes, such as Shish Kabob, are a great way to fill up on vegetables while keeping beef volume down. Be sure to mark your eight "splurge" meals on your PrescriptFit™ Calendar.

Something to Think About

If fish and beef contain no carbohydrate, why does beef contain 125 calories per ounce and fish only 25 calories per ounce? Fat! Remember: fat contains 9 calories per gram while protein and carbohydrate contain 4 calories per gram.

CATEGORIES OF BEEF AND CALORIES

Most people are familiar with beef cuts and marbleized fat in beef. When cattle are fed regular feed and have moderate marbleized fat, they produce "choice" cuts of beef. Those fed high grades of feed, usually corn, have more marbleized fat, producing "prime" cuts. Most people think prime cuts taste better since they contain more fat.

Highest fat cuts include:

- Rib-eye or Filet Mignon
- Sirloin
- T-bone
- Strip (sirloin)
- Porterhouse
- Tenderloin or Filet Mignon

Leaner cuts include round steak, roasts, and chuck. Ground beef is mixed with "parts" of other beef, usually fat scraps, used as fillers. Ground beef marked as "95 percent fat free" is very inaccurate.

All beef is at least 50 percent fat; therefore "percent fat" is a marketing gimmick that ends up falsely assuring you the product is not harmful to your health.

BOB OWEN'S BEEF RECIPES

SMOTHERED ROUND STEAK

2–3 round steaks
1 onions, chopped
1 green bell pepper, chopped
1 Knorr® bouillon cube, dissolved in
    1 cup water
1 bay leaf
¼ cup PrescriptFit™ Chicken Soup mixed in
    ¼ cup of water
Non-stick cooking spray
Salt
Cajun/Creole seasoning mix or black pepper

Dust the round steaks with Cajun/Creole seasoning mix or black pepper and salt. Lightly coat a large sauté pan with non-stick cooking spray and heat to medium-high. Brown the round steaks on both sides; remove and set aside. Add the onions and bell peppers to the same pan and sauté all ingredients for 1–2 minutes. Return the beef to the same pan. Add the bay leaf and the dissolved bouillon. Cover and cook for 15–20 minutes or until the bell peppers mute in color. Add the PrescriptFit™ Chicken soup to the sauce and mix until a gravy forms. Serve.

Sweet & Spicy Beef (may substitute chicken or pork)

1 lean beef steak (round steak, London broil or
  ask your butcher for a specialty lean cut)
¼ onion
¼ bell pepper
1 tablespoon mustard powder
2 packets Splenda®
3 tablespoons soy sauce
1 teaspoon horseradish
¼ cup green onions, chopped (tops and
  bottoms)
3–4 dashes Worcestershire sauce
¼ cup chopped parsley
Non-stick cooking spray
Black pepper or Cajun/Creole seasoning
  mix
Chili powder
Garlic powder
Salt

Marinate the beef in Worcestershire sauce
and salt. Heat a large sauté pan to high or
medium-high. Lightly coat the hot pan with
non-stick cooking spray. Rub the steak with
black pepper or Cajun/Creole seasoning on
both sides. Sear the steak in the pan, but do
not burn. Remove the steak and set to the side.

Add the onions, green onions, and bell
peppers to the pan. Cook for 2 minutes,
then add ½ cup of water. Add the remaining
ingredients and continue to cook for 20
minutes. Serve.

SKILLET STEAK IN WILD MUSHROOM & ROASTED GARLIC SAUCE

16 cloves garlic, unpeeled (for roasting)*
Coarse salt and freshly ground black pepper
1 ½ pounds top sirloin steaks, boneless, trimmed of fat
½ pound wild mushrooms
1 cup PrescriptFit™ Beef Soup mixed with 1 cup water
2 teaspoons fresh thyme leaves
Non-stick butter spray

Preheat oven to 375 degrees. Dry steaks thoroughly on paper towels and set aside.

Lightly coat a large skillet with nonstick cooking spray, heat over medium-high heat. Add mushrooms, and sauté quickly until lightly browned. Season with salt and pepper. Transfer to a side dish and reserve.

When the pan is almost smoking, add the steaks without crowding the pan. Sear steaks quickly on each side until nicely browned. Season with salt and pepper, reduce heat and continue to cook, covered, for 3 ½ minutes per side for medium rare. Remove steaks to a side dish and keep warm.

Discard all fat from skillet, and reduce juices to a glaze. Add PrescriptFit™ Beef Soup; simmer. Add mushrooms, garlic, thyme, and just heat through. Taste and correct the seasoning, adding a generous grinding of black pepper.

Slice each steak crosswise into small strips. Spoon sauce onto plate beside the steak, and serve at once.

*To Roast Garlic:

Place garlic cloves on a large piece of aluminum foil and sprinkle with salt and pepper.

Fold edges of foil over garlic and crimp to enclose completely.

Place the foil packet in the center of the oven, and roast for 30 minutes.

Open the foil and roast for an additional 10 minutes, or until lightly brown and tender.

Remove from the oven and let cool.

Carefully peel garlic, keeping the cloves whole, and set aside.

Beef and Vegetable Stew

1 lb. stew meat
½ onion
½ bell pepper
2 stalks celery, chopped
1 beef bouillon cube or one teaspoon of
    PrescriptFit™ Beef Soup powder
1 chicken bouillon cube or one teaspoon of
    PrescriptFit™ Chicken Soup powder
1 teaspoon minced garlic
1 bay leaf
1 teaspoon black pepper or Cajun/Creole
    seasoning mix
2–3 dashes of white pepper
1 teaspoon garlic powder
1 teaspoon thyme
1 teaspoon chili powder
¼ cup chopped parsley
¼ cup green onions
Non-stick cooking spray

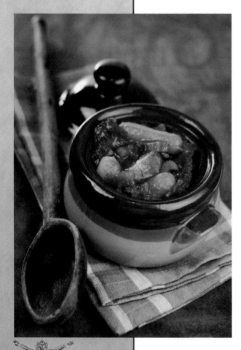

Lightly coat the bottom of a large soup pot with non-stick cooking spray and heat to medium-high. Season the meat with black pepper or Cajun/Creole seasoning, then brown for 3–5 minutes.

Add 3 cups of water and the remaining ingredients. Simmer for 25–35 minutes on medium heat. Serve.

PHASE 11 BEVERAGES

We recommend you save your beverages for your eight splurge meals (events) per month. For example, PrescriptFit™ shakes mixed with alcoholic beverages can help you limit your calorie consumption because the drinks are filling while supplying some of your amino acid daily dose recommendations.

BEVERAGES AS NUTRITION

Elimination of caloric (calorie containing) beverages is the single most substantial act you can take to minimize calories with any diet. We often consume beverages hurriedly and without much sensation of fullness or satiation. Seldom do we finish a beverage and say, "Wow, what a memorable experience." Therefore, caloric beverages are truly "empty" calories — empty nutrition and empty pleasure. Any and all diet (zero calorie) beverages are allowed with the Plan.

Milk is the only caloric beverage of sufficient nutrient value to consider using as a nutritious beverage. However, whole milk contains over 50 percent saturated fat by dry weight; 2 percent milk is about 35 percent saturated fat by dry weight; skim milk contains about

Reminder:
- Continue 6–8 or more PrescriptFit™ amino acid doses per day.
- Use PrescriptFit™ shakes or soups before or with meals.
- Use foods from Phases 2–8.
- Use Phase 11 beverages for splurges ONLY.
- Take a multi-vitamin supplement.
- Drink 5 cups of water or calorie-free beverage daily.

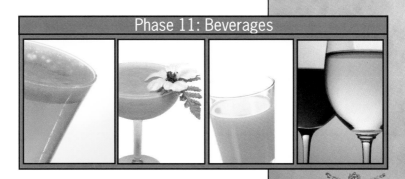

Phase 11: Beverages

10 percent saturated fat. Only powdered nonfat milk is completely devoid of dangerous saturated fat. Most people are not willing to put up with the taste of powdered nonfat milk for routine consumption. Milk tastes good because of the saturated fat. Saturated fat is "sticky." It sticks to your arteries like milk sticks to your lip or butter to your hand. Saturated fat has adverse effects on blood vessel and insulin function. Therefore, if milk must be consumed, skim or nonfat milk are the best options.

Non-fat milk contains protein and complex carbohydrates. It also contains substantial amounts of calcium. Dietary calcium has been associated with weight loss and health benefits. Calcium directly suppresses cytokine production in fat cells and the liver. PrescriptFit™ amino acid shakes and soups contain nonfat milk solids with 100 percent of adult daily calcium requirements. No extra calcium supplements are needed with five or more PrescriptFit doses per day.

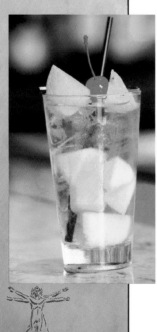

Alcoholic beverages have demonstrated protection against heart attack and stroke. However, what dose of alcohol provides best protection is unclear. Due to calorie considerations and toxic effects of high alcohol doses, alcoholic beverages are placed in the "splurge" meal categories — eight meals (events) per month.

The Amino Solution
©2009 Stanford A. Owen, MD

Beverage Myths

The notion that juice is a "healthy" beverage is badly misplaced. Concentrated sugar is not healthy in any form — including juices. Many juices have added sugar or have been concentrated to increase sweetness. Juices fortified with calcium or vitamins have far less calcium or vitamins than can be obtained from a non-caloric vitamin or mineral supplement.

Milk has been promoted as nature's most "perfect food." It is — if you're an infant animal with a growing nervous system that needs fat for growth. However, the saturated fat in milk is harmful to adult arteries.

Sport drinks contain sugar and calories, and they contribute to obesity and insulin resistance. Avoid sports drinks.

The worst myth is "diet" drinks that contain saccharin or aspartame are harmful. Data about harm are virtually non-existent while safety data on these products are abundant. Compared to sugar in soft drinks, artificial sweeteners are infinitely less harmful.

Remember that it takes one mile of walking to burn 100 calories!

The Centers for Disease Control notes the #1 cause of preventable cancer is not cigarettes, but obesity. The #1 contributor to obesity is consuming caloric beverages.

Beverage	Calories/Ounce	Walking distance required to burn those calories
Diet drinks	0	0
Soft drinks	12	1.5 miles per 12-ounce can
Beer	12	1.5 miles per 12-ounce can
Juice	20	1.5 miles per 8-ounce glass
Milk	20	1.5 miles per 8-ounce glass
Wine	20	1 mile per 4- to 6-ounce glass
Liquor	60	1 mile per 1 ½-ounce shot
Liqueur	100–150	2 miles per shot

The Amino Solution
©2009 Stanford A. Owen, MD

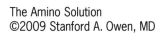

Bob Owen's Beverages Recipes

Each of the beverage recipes makes two drinks.
Place all ingredients in a blender, fill with ice,
blend, and **Enjoy!**

PrescriptFit™ Pina Colada

> 4 scoops vanilla PrescriptFit™
> 1 cup water
> 1 teaspoon coconut extract (McCormick®
>   flavorings)
> 2 jiggers rum
> ⅛ teaspoon cinnamon

PrescriptFit™ Strawberry Daiquiri

> 4 scoops vanilla PrescriptFit™
> 1 cup cold water
> 1 tablespoon Jell-O® Sugar Free Strawberry
>   Gelatin (or 1 cup fresh strawberries)
> 2 jiggers rum
> ⅛ teaspoon of pumpkin pie spice

PrescriptFit™ Banana Banshee

> 4 scoops of vanilla PrescriptFit™
> 1 cup water
> ¼ teaspoon banana extract
> ¼ teaspoon rum extract
> 2 jiggers rum
> ⅛ teaspoon cinnamon

PrescriptFit™ Tropical Fruit Delight

> 4 scoops vanilla PrescriptFit™
> 1 cup water
> 1–2 teaspoons Crystal Light®
> Tropical Fruit (2 tsp. is quite tart)
> 2 jiggers rum

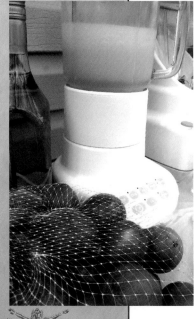

PrescriptFit™ Calypso Fudge

- 4 scoops chocolate Lactose Free PrescriptFit™
- 1 cup water
- 1 jigger Kahlua® liqueur (or 1 teaspoon granulated instant coffee for less calories)
- 1 teaspoon Hershey's® pure unsweetened cocoa powder
- 2 jiggers rum
- ⅛ teaspoon cinnamon

PrescriptFit™ Cappuccino Kahlua® Delight

- 4 scoops chocolate Lactose Free PrescriptFit™
- 1 cup water
- 1 teaspoon of coffee extract
- 1 tablespoon Kahlua® liqueur
- 2 jiggers rum

PrescriptFit™ Mango Daiquiri

- 4 scoops vanilla PrescriptFit ™
- 1 cup water
- 1 teaspoon mango extract or 1 cup fresh mango
- 1 teaspoon Crystal Light® tropical fruit drink mix
- 2 jiggers rum

PrescriptFit™ Crème de Lite

- 4 scoops vanilla PrescriptFit™
- 1 cup water
- 2 jiggers Crème de Menthe
- ½ teaspoon mint extract
- 2 jiggers rum or coconut rum (for more tropical taste).

GINGER — MANAGING LIQUID CALORIES

Ginger and her coworkers enjoyed meeting after work at the pub just around the corner from office. Being single, Ginger tended to join the group two or three evenings a week rather than going home to an empty apartment.

A problem Ginger didn't count on (literally) involved the calories she consumed sharing pitchers of beer (plus the occasional high-fat appetizer plate) on such a frequent basis. Ginger had gained 40 pounds in the past year. She attributed her more frequent drinking with her friends to needing to relieve some of the "stress" at work and to being lonely.

I suggested Ginger save the drinking for "TGIFs" once her weight was back under control. I strongly recommended she exchange the time at the pub for time at the gym, perhaps getting some of her friends to join with her. Exercise helps with mental health as much as physical health. Moreover, exercise has been shown to significantly decrease the "stress" Ginger complained of from her job.

Ginger met Buddy later that year at the gym. She is now married, and has a baby boy. She feels and looks great and finds TGIF more than adequate to quench her partying soul and stay connected with her friends.

CASE STUDY

Phase 12 Dairy

Dairy is added in the final PrescriptFit™ Phases since dairy products are easy to over-consume. Dairy can be harmful or healthful, depending on the type and amount consumed.

Dairy Nutrition

Most dairy products are now available in nonfat varieties. Dairy products that would traditionally contain sugar, like ice cream, can be made with artificial sweeteners and nonfat milk, decreasing fat and calories. Dairy should be considered a condiment to enhance flavors in Food Phases 1–11 or as a stand-alone treat for dessert.

Dairy products made from whole milk contain about 50 percent of calories from fat, 30 percent from carbohydrate, and 20 percent from protein. The fat is harmful saturated fat. Non-fat milk contains about 60 percent complex carbohydrate and 40 percent protein (whey).

Dairy Myths

We've all grown up believing the myth that milk is essential for growth and development after infancy. However, we are the only species

Reminder:
- Continue 6–8 or more PrescriptFit™ amino acid doses per day.
- Use PrescriptFit™ shakes or soups before or with meals.
- Use foods from Phases 2–8.
- Use Phase 12 for splurges ONLY (except for nonfat cheese and yogurt.
- Take a multi-vitamin supplement.
- Drink 5 cups of water or calorie-free beverage daily.

The three main sources of harmful saturated fat in modern diets are:
- Fried Foods
- Dairy Products
- Fatty meats

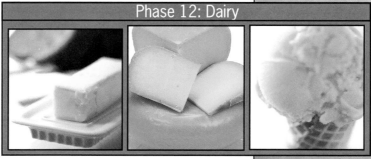

Phase 12: Dairy

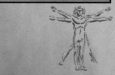

The Amino Solution
©2009 Stanford A. Owen, MD

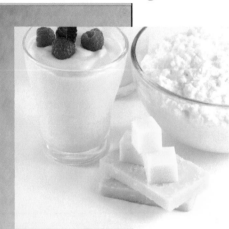

that consumes milk after infancy. Certainly calcium is beneficial for bone density, especially during the growth spurt in adolescent children. But calcium is readily available from many sources of less-fattening foods, such as vegetables.

The PrescriptFit™ product dosing is designed to provide enough calcium to the daily diet without the need for extra calcium supplementation — about 1,500 mg/day.

Clearly those items with the most fat have the most calories. Those with the most calories are also most harmful to arteries and abnormal metabolism.

How far would you need to walk in a month to pay back one glass of milk per day? A whopping 44 miles! Avoid milk.

DAIRY FOOD	CALORIES PER OUNCE	CALORIES PER TYPICAL SERVING
Yogurt (regular)	50	200
Yogurt (nonfat)	25	100
Sour cream (regular)	50	200
Sour cream (nonfat)	30	100
Cream cheese (regular)	75	200
Cream cheese (nonfat)	30	100
Cheese (regular)	100	400
Cheese (nonfat)	25	200
Ice cream (regular)	125–150	500–1000
Milk	20	160
Cream	75	400

The Amino Solution
©2009 Stanford A. Owen, MD

DAIRY CATEGORIES

- Milk
- Buttermilk
- Cream
- Cheese
- Cottage cheese
- Yogurt
- Ice cream
- Sour cream
- Cream cheese
- Whipped creams

> ### *Dosing*
> *Only nonfat cottage cheese, nonfat cheese, and nonfat yogurt are allowed in unlimited doses; all other dairy items are for splurge meals ONLY.*

DAIRY DOSING ADVICE

Only nonfat cottage cheese, nonfat cheese, and nonfat yogurt are allowed in unlimited doses since their calorie content is equivalent to seafood. They may even be used in place of seafood or poultry as a main dish or "entrée" meal component. Non-fat sour cream and cream cheese should be used sparingly as a condiment. Ice cream and cream dishes should be used only on "splurge" meals. The chart on the next page outlines specific dosing advice.

Non-fat cheese is equivalent to seafood or poultry and may be used as replacement for those choices. Use regular cheese only for splurge meals.

Wilson — Victim of Dairy Overload

Wilson weighed 550 pounds when he came to our clinic, claiming he didn't eat "anything." On interview, I found he didn't "eat anything" indeed. He drank everything — two gallons of whole milk per day and a liter of cola — that's about 6,000 calories per day of milk alone. I calculated he should weigh even more!

Marketed as a "health food" for over 50 years, dairy is a major culprit in the epidemic of obesity. One glass of milk at 150 calories, seven days per week, four weeks per month, and 52 weeks per year equals 54,750 calories or 16 pounds per year. Worth it? Maybe.

Perhaps those 54,750 calories would be better enjoyed on a Splurge?

CASE STUDY

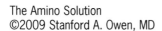

DAIRY DOSING ADVICE

Cottage Cheese (non fat)

Use in place of seafood or poultry for a "meat" selection (but not until after you have reached Food Phase 12 in sequence). Non-fat cottage cheese is almost pure protein at 25 calories per ounce. You can mix it with fresh or canned fruit for flavor or use Splenda® if you want a "sweet" taste. As with fish and poultry, you can eat unlimited amounts of nonfat cottage cheese.

Yogurt

Yogurt, preferably non-fat or low-fat yogurt, may be used as a main serving or a dessert. It is especially tasty as a dessert with fresh fruit or mixed with nuts. Watch your serving size carefully, as it is easy to over-consume yogurt.

Sour Cream and Cream Cheese

These two condiments should be used on vegetables and selected meat dishes. Non-fat varieties are available; however, careful dosing is suggested.

Cream, Cheese, and Ice Cream (Splurge ONLY)

Use these items only for your eight "splurge" meals per month. At 100-150 calories per ounce, they have the same caloric content and saturated fat as beef or pork. They can cause serious harm to those with diabetes, hypertension, and heart disease.

Non-fat Cheese

Non-fat cheese is equivalent to seafood or poultry and may be used as replacement for those choices.

Non-fat Whipped Cream

You may use the non-fat variety on desserts, puddings, etc. Avoid the full-fat version.

Milk, Buttermilk, Cream

Avoid these dairy products due to the tendency to over consume excess calories and fat.

BOB OWEN'S DAIRY RECIPES

LEMON YOGURT

> 1–2 cups low-calorie/fat-free vanilla yogurt
> 1 lemon
> 2 packets Splenda®

Cut the pulp out of the lemon and discard the white core and the peel. Mix the lemon pulp with the Splenda® until completely dissolved. Add a sprinkle of water if not completely dissolved. Mix with the vanilla yogurt. Serve.

SQUASH SOUP

> 3–4 sliced yellow squash
> Non-stick cooking spray
> 1 onion, chopped finely
> 1 cup chicken broth or dissolved bouillon
> 1 cup fat-free half & half
> 2 tablespoons fat-free butter spray or
>   Benecol® spread
> ¼ cup chopped green onions

Lightly coat the bottom of a soup pot with non-stick cooking spray and heat to medium-high. Add the onions and squash, and cook until the onions begin to brown. Add the chicken broth and continue to cook for 5 minutes. Pour the soup into a blender, and blend until the consistency is smooth. Pour the mixture back into the pot. Add the half & half and the butter spray or Benecol® spread. Add the green onions and serve.

The Amino Solution
©2009 Stanford A. Owen, MD

Jalapeño Cream Cheese Dip

1 cup nonfat or low-fat cream cheese
2–3 jalapeno peppers, with seeds removed
    (spicy part of the pepper)
2 tablespoons fat-free half & half
1–2 dashes chili powder
1–2 dashes salt
1–2 dashes paprika

Mince jalapeno peppers. Mix all ingredients together until it's a creamy dip consistency. Enjoy as a dip for raw vegetables.

Chocolate Cream Pie

1 cup pecans, crushed
2 tablespoons Smart Balance® or
    Benecol® spread
10 scoops PrescriptFit™ Lactose Free
    Chocolate
2 cups of water
Sugar-free, fat-free whipped topping

Mix pecans with Smart Balance® or Benecol® spread. Spread mixture over bottom of pie pan to form a shell.

Stir PrescriptFit™ mix with water, adding "dribbles" of water at a time while stirring until texture is that of a creamy pudding.

Pour the pudding over pecan mixture, and cover with whipped topping.

PHASE 13 BAKED GOODS AND OTHER STARCHY FOODS

This Phase includes some obvious starchy foods, such as potatoes, rice, bread, pasta, and baked goods. It also includes starchy vegetables, such as corn, peas, and parsnips.

STARCHY FOODS AND NUTRITION

Starchy foods — including starchy vegetables and baked goods — are reserved for the final Phase of the Plan because these foods are most likely to induce symptoms and weight gain. The reasons are clear:

- Baked goods are higher in calories per ounce compared to foods in Food Phases 1–8.

- Baked goods contain refined carbohydrates and fat (usually saturated or "trans" vegetable fat) that is quickly absorbed — the so-called "glycemic" effect that promotes insulin release, insulin resistance, and cytokine production.

- Baked goods are very tasty because of the sugar-fat combination, and are easily over consumed. Yet they are not filling, leading to even more consumption.

Reminder:

- Continue 6–8 or more PrescriptFit™ amino acid doses per day.
- Use PrescriptFit™ shakes or soups before or with meals.
- Use foods from Phases 2–8.
- Use Phase 13 foods for splurges ONLY.
- Take a multi-vitamin supplement.
- Drink 5 cups of water or calorie-free beverage daily.

Phase 13: Baked Goods/Other Starchy Foods

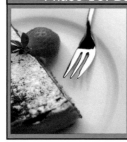
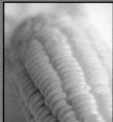
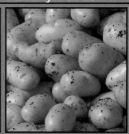

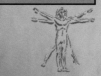

> ***Dosing— Splurge Only!***
> *All Food Phase 13 foods are used as "splurge" meals —*
> *up to eight per month. Use the PrescriptFit™ Calendar to*
> *mark "splurge" meals.*

- Starchy vegetables are considerably lower in calories and fat than most baked goods, but can be over-consumed.

BAKED GOODS MYTHS

Carbohydrates, or "carbs," are the talk of the decade. As the obesity epidemic and obesity-related diseases, such as diabetes, have exploded in prevalence, we needed something to blame. The Atkins diet, and similar high fat, high protein diets, made "carb" a four-letter word.

The fact is controlled intake of baked goods that are low in fat is no more harmful than any other food item. The challenge is to control your portions of baked items. That's not always easy to do, especially when you're eating out or buying commercially produced items. For example, the muffins available in the store are usually so large one muffin can easily contain 1,000 calories. The best way to control baked good calories is to use these items on "splurge" meals and no more than eight meals per month.

CATEGORIES AND CALORIES OF STARCHY VEGETABLES

While high in calories, starchy vegetables are not all bad. Consider, for example:

- One cup of starchy vegetables equals only two ounces of beef or pork — a good caloric value.

- Two cups of beans — enough to cover an entire plate at 400 calories — is less than the calories of one donut (150 calories/oz) at 500 calories.

Starchy Vegetable	Calories per cup
Potatoes	125
Corn	150
Dried beans	200
Rice	200

- Starchy vegetables are loaded with fiber and vitamins.

Categories and Calories of Baked Goods

Baked Good	Calories per ounce	Distance to walk to pay back calories
Bread (white, whole wheat, rolls, bagels, English muffins)	80	1.5 miles for 1 slice of bread (150 cal.)
Muffins, corn bread, biscuits, pretzels, baked chips	100	6–8 miles for the average muffin
Cereals (cold or hot)	110	4 miles for a bowl of cereal plus milk
Pastries (donuts, Danish, croissants, crackers, cookies, cake)	125	5 miles per donut; 10 miles per large cookie; 5–7 miles per slice of cake
Pies (all types), corn and potato chips, chocolate	150	6–10 miles per slice of pie; 3 miles per 2-ounce bag of chips.

Before you indulge, remember the basic principles upon which all diets are designed: People lose weight when they consume fewer calories than they need for metabolism in the organs and through physical activity. Baked goods may taste good, but they produce minimal satiation or fullness compared to

Consider this:

Muffins sold at airport deli stands average 10-12 ounces per muffin (or 1,000 calories!!).

A large piece of pecan pie will require up to 10 miles of walking payback!

The Amino Solution
©2009 Stanford A. Owen, MD

⌐ Section B: Diving In... ⌐

The caloric content of most baked goods is as high or higher than beef or pork, is far less satiating or filling, and will contribute to:

- Excess insulin secretion
- insulin resistance
- excess cytokine production

high protein foods. So ask yourself: Are these calories worth it or not?

Baked Goods are the items most likely to "jump out" and grab you unexpectedly at social events, work site break rooms, or with addictive binge eating. By marking your calendar when you indulge unexpectedly in starchy foods, and by removing a planned splurge meal, you'll be able to evaluate your experience. Was that Little Debbie® really worth removing the steak or ice cream from the calendar?

BOB OWEN'S STARCHY FOOD RECIPES

BLACK BEAN DIP (SERVED WITH BAKED TORTILLA CHIPS)

½ lb. dry black beans (or 1 ¾ cups canned cooked black beans)
1 1/ cups canned mild Rotel® original diced tomatoes and chilies
1 tablespoon fresh garlic, minced
1 large bouillon cube
1 bay leaf
½ onion, chopped
½ bell pepper, chopped
½ stalk celery, finely chopped
Non-stick cooking spray
½ teaspoon salt
½ teaspoon garlic powder
½ teaspoon dried thyme
½ teaspoon white pepper
½ teaspoon black pepper
1 teaspoon chili powder
½ cup chopped fresh parsley
½ cup chopped green onion
¼ cup chopped cilantro

Cook beans as instructed on package, except add 1 large bouillon cube. Lightly coat a separate sauté pan with non-stick cooking spray, heat to medium-high, and sauté onions, bell peppers, garlic, bay leaf, and celery for 10-15 minutes. Remove the bay leaf and add sauté mixture to the beans. Add fresh, chopped cilantro and other ingredients. Puree the mixture. Finish with chopped green onions and chopped parsley. May be served warm or cold.

Pasta Fagoli

    4 cups chicken broth
    1 cup canned navy beans
    1 ½ cups rigatoni
    1 bay leaf
    1 teaspoon garlic
    1 teaspoon black pepper
    ½ salt
    ½ teaspoon garlic powder
    ½ teaspoon sage
    ½ teaspoon oregano
    ½ teaspoon basil
    ¼ cup chopped parsley

Bring broth to a boil. Add rigatoni pasta. Cook until tender. Add the remaining ingredients except parsley. Cook for 10 minutes on medium heat. With a spoon, mash a few of the beans until the sauce thickens. Add salt and pepper to taste and finish with parsley.

Corn Stew

    3 bouillon cubes (dissolved in 3 cups water)
        or 3 teaspoons PrescriptFit™ Chicken
        Soup
    ½ onion, chopped
    ½ bell pepper, chopped
    2 celery stalks, chopped
    1 bay leaf
    3 ½ cups canned whole kernel corn
    1 tablespoon garlic, chopped
    1 tablespoon fat-free butter spray or
        Benecol® spread

The Amino Solution
©2009 Stanford A. Owen, MD

2 tablespoons fat-free half & half
Non-stick cooking spray
Black pepper
Garlic powder
Thyme
Chili powder
Salt
¼ cup green onions
¼ cup parsley

Lightly coat the bottom of a large stew or soup pot with non-stick cooking spray. Heat to medium-high and sauté onions, bell peppers, celery, garlic, and corn for 5-8 minutes. Add broth and bay leaf. Simmer for 10 minutes. Add remaining ingredients. Season & cook for 8-10 minutes more. Finish with green onions and parsley.

POTATO SOUP

3 medium potatoes (4 oz each),
    peeled and diced
4 cups chicken broth
½ onion, chopped
½ bell pepper, chopped
1 stalk celery, chopped
1 bay leaf
1 teaspoon garlic powder
1 teaspoon thyme
2-3 dashes dried basil
1 teaspoon dried sage
1 teaspoon chili powder
½ cup of fat-free half and half
2 teaspoons Benecol® spread
¼ cup green onions
¼ cup parsley

Place all ingredients, except the green onions and parsley, into a large stew pot. Bring to a boil. Reduce heat to a simmer. Cook for 40 minutes. Mash mixture until thickening begins. Add water if the mixture is too thick. Finish with green onions and parsley. Serve.

Onion Peas

3 cups canned baby peas (not bright green
or large)
½ onion, chopped
1 tablespoon fat-free butter spray or
Benecol® spread
1 teaspoon black pepper or Cajun/Creole
seasoning mix
Several dashes of salt
Non-stick cooking spray

Lightly coat a small pot with non-stick
cooking spray. Heat to medium-high. Saute
the onion for 3-8 minutes. Add remaining
ingredients and continue to cook for 2-4
minutes. Serve.

Smothered Black-Eyed Peas with Rice

3 ½ cups canned black-eyed peas
1 onion, chopped
1 bell pepper, chopped
2 cups cooked rice
1 cup chicken broth
1 bay leaf
Non-stick cooking spray
1 teaspoon black pepper or Cajun/Creole
seasoning mix
1 teaspoon garlic powder
1 teaspoon thyme
1 teaspoon salt
¼ cup chopped green onions
¼ cup chopped parsley

Lightly coat a large sauté pan with non-stick
cooking spray and heat to medium-high. Add
the onions and bell peppers, and sauté for
4-8 minutes. Add the remaining ingredients
(except the parsley, green onions, and rice),
and cook for 10-15 minutes. Add green onions
and parsley. Mix in the cooked rice and serve.

The Amino Solution
©2009 Stanford A. Owen, MD

NOTES

_____

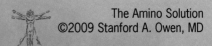

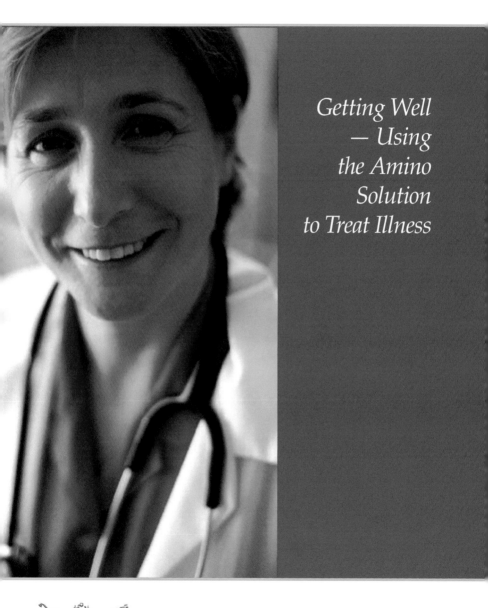

*Getting Well
— Using
the Amino
Solution
to Treat Illness*

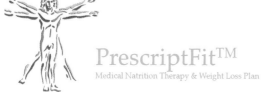

PrescriptFit™
Medical Nutrition Therapy & Weight Loss Plan

THE AMINO SOLUTION
TABLE OF CONTENTS

Section C: Getting Well — Using the Amino Solution to Treat Illness

The Amino Solution was developed as a way to help treat illness and chronic symptoms that keep you from feeling your best. The concept of Medical Nutrition Therapy (MNT) is about:

> **Improving your quality of life on a very basic level of wellness** — a first step toward enhancing other areas of anyone's life. It's hard to do the things you need to improve your education, your work situation, or your relationships if you just don't feel well.

> **Participating with your physician** to get the best quality medical care you can; that means you and your physician working together to diagnose and treat disease AND to measure response to treatment.

> **"Fitting" treatment for illness to the individual.** Each person's health changes as diet, age, illness, medication, or life events change. What makes your body perform at its best may be very different from those around you and at different times and during different circumstances you encounter in life.

> **Learning that disease and diet are intimately connected** AND exactly how you can balance that connection to feel better. As you introduce each new Food Phase you discover what, how, and when your symptoms improve or worsen.

The Amino Solution's Medical Nutrition Therapy stresses:

- Actively working with your doctor
- Using nutrition change to help treat a variety of medical conditions
- Discovering for yourself exactly what level or type of lifestyle change makes YOU feel better
- Measuring response REGULARLY to nutrition change

The Amino Solution
©2009 Stanford A. Owen, MD

Chapter 8: The Link Between Diet & Illness

On a global scale, quality of life is defined as, "...a broad ranging concept, incorporating in a complex way individuals' physical health, psychological state, level of independence, social relationships, personal beliefs, and their relationships to salient features of the environment...quality of life is subjective, includes both positive and negative facets of life and is multi-dimensional."

[The World Health Organization Quality of Life Group, 1995, p. 1405]

Quality of Life and the Amino Solution

On a personal level (apart from income, social, family, and cultural issues), how we might rate our individual quality of life tends to have a lot to do with:

> Eating things that taste good and avoiding digestive problems, such as GERD (acid reflux) and irritable bowel syndrome

> Avoiding chronic illness, such as diabetes mellitus, hypertension, hyperlipidemia, insulin resistant syndrome (IRS or metabolic syndrome), steatosis (fatty liver)

> Feeling energetic without suffering the overall fatigue of fibromyalgia or the debilitating sadness of depression

> Moving without pain and/or swelling often associated with migraine headaches and arthritis as well as back, knee, and joint pain

Clinical experience with PrescriptFit™ for over 10 years has shown that MNT positively augments treatment for disorders that seriously compromise elements of daily quality of life.

The Amino Solution
©2009 Stanford A. Owen, MD

～ Chapter 8: The Link Between Diet & Illness ～

> Enjoying sex instead of worrying about problems with libido, sexual dysfunction, or infertility

> Increasing the odds of living longer by minimizing the risk of heart disease and stroke

> Breathing easy without suffering shortness of breath or asthma and allergies

> Sleeping soundly and regularly by controlling sleep apnea and insomnia

From our 10 years' clinical experience with PrescriptFit™, we've found that MNT positively augments treatment for these disorders that seriously compromise these most basic elements of daily quality of life.

This chapter includes specific information about a variety of disease/symptom categories positively impacted by MNT.

Disease/Symptom Questionnaires are located following each topic to measure response after each Food Phase or every four weeks. These questionnaires also appear at the back of your PrescriptFit™ Calendar.

Medical textbooks cite MNT as the first line of treatment for many diseases, including:

- Acid reflux (GERD)
- Diabetes
- Migraines
- High cholesterol
- High blood pressure
- Metabolic syndrome (IRS)
- Irritable bowel syndrome
- Sleep apnea
- Steatosis (fatty liver)

Use the chart on the next page to quickly access how to approach using MNT for those diseases or symptoms that "fit" for you.

*Section C: Getting Well... *

QUALITY OF LIFE (QoL) MEASURES AND MNT TREATMENT			
Diseases/Symptoms Impacting QoL Measures	MNT = First-line	MNT = Adjunct	MNT Supervision*
HEALTHY DIGESTION			
• Acid Reflux (GERD)	X		
• Irritable Bowel Syndrome (IBS)	X		
RENEWED ENERGY			
• Fatigue		X	
• Fibromyalgia		X	
• Depression		X	
PAIN FREEDOM/MOBILITY			
• Migraine	X		
• Arthritis		X	X
• Back, Knee, and Joint Pain		X	
• Edema (Swelling)		X	
IMPROVED SEXUALITY			
• Low Libido		X	
• Sexual Dysfunction		X	
• Infertility		X	
GOOD NIGHT'S REST			
• Sleep Apnea/Snoring	X		
• Insomnia		X	
WELL-MANAGED CHRONIC ILLNESS			
• Diabetes Mellitus	X		X
• Hypertension	X	X	X
• Hyperlipidemia	X	X	X
• Metabolic Syndrome (IRS)	X	X	
• Steatosis (fatty liver)	X	X	X
• Dyspnea (breathlessness)		X	X
• Congestive Heart Failure		X	X
• Angina Pectoris		X	X
• Asthma		X	X

* WARNING: MNT REQUIRES CLOSE PHYSICIAN SUPERVISION: YOUR DOCTOR MAY WANT YOU TO DISCONTINUE CERTAIN MEDICATIONS QUICKLY IF YOUR DISEASE SYMPTOMS SUBSIDE TO AVOID CRITICAL PROBLEMS WITH BLOOD PRESSURE OR CARDIAC FUNCTION.

≈ Chapter 8: The Link Between Diet & Illness ≈

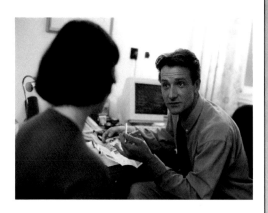

YOU, YOUR DOCTOR, AND THE AMINO SOLUTION

The Amino Solution — combining Medical Nutrition Therapy and PrescriptFit™ products — is designed to help you and your doctor treat diet-responsive disease and measure results. Diet-responsive illnesses are those that positively improve when treatment includes a change in the way you eat. Every diet-responsive medical condition has specific **signs, symptoms, or measures.**

> **A sign** is something you can easily see — An increase/decrease in weight, change in waist size, swelling, changes in skin coloration (pink/ gray).

> **A symptom** is something you feel — Fatigue, shortness of breath, snoring, pain, sadness, worry

> **A measure** is something you learn from a lab text or exam procedure — Blood pressure, blood sugar count, or cholesterol level

You may have several medical conditions present at the same time that require taking a variety of medications, even some that counteract the side effects of others. Ask your doctor to help you learn to measure each medical condition independently to better understand whether or not what you eat contributes to the problem.

Remember, a diet is something very personal. Who we are, how we feel, and how we look in size and shape are the results of what we eat, our eating habits as well as our lifestyle. If you want to change the way you FEEL, you need to find a way to change your "diet" to what your body needs to make you feel better.

With MNT, you use the number of doses of amino acids, the information you collect about how you feel, and the flexible Food Phases to design the "diet" that works best to feel better from now on.

The PrescriptFit™ Disease/Symptom Questionnaires and scoring systems are based on Dr. Owen's clinical experience from the past 10 years. These results are important primarily for what they might mean for you, and secondly for helping your doctor treat your illness.

CHAPTER 9: MNT AS FIRST-LINE TREATMENT

MNT can be used as a first-line treatment for managing symptoms associated with:

- Acid reflux (GERD)
- Diabetes
- Migraines
- High cholesterol
- High blood pressure
- Metabolic syndrome (IRS)
- Irritable bowel syndrome
- Sleep apnea
- Steatosis (fatty liver)

Key to this treatment is keeping track of the symptoms you have, how severe they might be, and how they might change as you follow the PrescriptFit™ Plan. You may notice that symptoms lessen significantly in the first few phases of the Plan, but return quickly when you get to the later phases or cut back on your amino acid doses.

Following the MNT Plan also means keeping track of what medications you take (both those prescribed by your doctor and those sold "over the counter") AND how often you take them. You may find that you will no longer need to take many of these medications OR take them nearly as often by following the MNT Plan.

Measuring the symptom changes you experience will give you the DATA you need to know how to fit MNT to you. The flexibility and creativity built into the Plan gives you the POWER to make that "fit" a creative, long-term solution to feeling better.

WARNING: Never change how much or how often you take any physician-prescribed medication without consulting your doctor.

The Amino Solution
©2009 Stanford A. Owen, MD

Acid Reflux Disease (GERD):
Dyspepsia; Heartburn; Peptic Ulcers

What is Acid Reflux?

Acid reflux or GERD occurs when acid from the stomach flows backward in the "swallowing tube" or esophagus. Typically, this happens because the muscle (sphincter) that keeps the lower end of the esophagus closed once food/liquid passes through to the stomach "relaxes" more than normal. This "reflux" often causes stomach pain, heartburn, indigestion, and/or bloating; sometimes, people experience chest pain or difficulty swallowing as a result. Left untreated, GERD can cause serious damage to the esophagus.

What Causes GERD?

Physicians really don't know why reflux occurs more in some people than others. One cause can be mechanical — a hiatal hernia (dislocation of the stomach through the "hiatus" of the diaphragm and into the chest) allows acid to penetrate the esophagus. "Stress" causes excess acid secretion, which can make the reflux more likely and more severe. Some medications (such as those often prescribed for arthritis) can dissolve the stomach's mucous lining, allowing damaging acid to "eat away" at the stomach. Finally, we know that a bacteria named "H. Pylori" damages the protective mucous barrier and directly inflames the stomach lining.

All four mechanisms — mechanical, stress, medications, and bacteria — may be present. In addition, the interrelationship of obesity, diet, and GERD is complex and hard to define.

Did you know?

1. GERD is the most common ailment worldwide.
2. Antacid medication is the #1 selling class of medication.
3. The incidence of GERD has steadily increased with worldwide obesity.

If these mechanisms can cause GERD, why do symptoms often disappear after only six weeks of a Medical Nutrition Therapy Plan? The answer is: we don't know!

⌒ Chapter 9: MNT as First-Line Treatment ⌒

What Role Might Cytokine Imbalance Play?

One theory is that fat cell-produced cytokines influence acid secretion, inflammation, and the ability to move food/liquid through the digestive system. When cytokine-producing diets change to cytokine-balancing diets, these functions improve.

What Results Could I Expect with MNT?

In my clinic, 67 percent of all patients at initial evaluation use some type of antacid medication for symptom relief. Within three months of beginning the PrescriptFit™ MNT Plan, 87 percent no longer suffer from GERD symptoms and can discontinue taking antacid medication.

How Can I Measure Symptom Change on the Plan?

First, you need to be clear about what symptoms of GERD you might have. Next, you want to have a measurement of how severe each symptom is for you. This will give you a "baseline" to compare with future measurements. Most importantly, talk with your doctor at each regular visit about your symptoms and how they might change using the PrescriptFit™ Plan.

As with any medical condition, treatment for GERD often involves taking medications to reduce symptoms. With PrescriptFit™, you may find that as your symptoms lessen, you will need to take less medication OR perhaps discontinue your medications entirely. If you are taking prescription medicines, talk to you doctor about when and how to cut down on what you take BEFORE you make any changes.

You (and your doctor) won't know how the Amino Solution is helping you without a way to measure progress.

The Amino Solution
©2009 Stanford A. Owen, MD

Section C: Getting Well...

WHAT DO I NEED TO DO?

1. Check each symptom you are currently experiencing in the Disease/Symptom Questionnaire below.
2. Grade the level of discomfort you have on a scale from 0-10 (with "0" being no symptom at all to a "10" being severe discomfort).
3. Be sure to check the symptoms and grade your level of discomfort AGAIN at the end of each Food Phase or every four weeks.
4. Check each medication you currently take for GERD and how often you take it. If you're taking over-the-counter antacids, be sure to record how much you're taking at the end of each Food Phase or every four weeks.
5. Take the results with you to your next doctor's appointment. Talk about how you're feeling and whether or not you still need any prescription medications for GERD.

ACID REFLUX (GERD) DISEASE/SYMPTOM QUESTIONNAIRE

Symptom Experience	Level of Discomfort
HEARTBURN	None Severe 0 1 2 3 4 5 6 7 8 9 10
PAIN IN PIT OF STOMACH	None Severe 0 1 2 3 4 5 6 7 8 9 10
FOOD/LIQUID IN MOUTH DURING SLEEP	None Nightly 0 1 2 3 4 5 6 7 8 9 10
BLOATING AFTER MEALS	None Daily 0 1 2 3 4 5 6 7 8 9 10

GERD Medications Used:
Circle those used and frequency as indicated below.

OVER-THE-COUNTER ANTACIDS (MAALOX™, TUMS™, ETC.)	Daily >2X/week >2X/month

PRESCRIPTION MEDICATIONS (CIRCLE ALL TAKEN ONCE A WEEK OR MORE)

Nexium	Pepcid	Propulsid	Prilosec
Prevacid	Tagamet	Zantac	
Protonix	Axid	Reglan	

Other (list) _____

* WARNING: NEVER DISCONTINUE A PHYSICIAN-PRESCRIBED MEDICATION WITHOUT CONSULTING YOUR DOCTOR

⌇ Chapter 9: MNT as First-Line Treatment ⌇

DIABETES MELLITUS
(ADULT ONSET OR TYPE II)

What is Diabetes Mellitus?

Diabetes mellitus results from your pancreas being unable to produce enough insulin to act on the "sugar" content in your bloodstream. Diabetes is defined as a fasting (12-hour fast) blood glucose (known as FPG) of 126 mg/dl or greater or a glucose level of 200 mg/dl or greater after a meal. A "pre-diabetes" condition exists when the fasting blood sugar is 110 mg/dl or above.

What Causes Diabetes?

Diabetes occurs when the pancreas does not produce sufficient insulin, which is a hormone essential for protein, fats, and sugars (glucose) to enter cells for growth and repair or energy production. When cells become "resistant" to the action of insulin (due to diet, lack of exercise, and genetic factors), cells "think" they are starving and send messages to the pancreas to produce more insulin (which is still ineffective). As a result, the pancreas becomes exhausted from chronic overproduction of insulin.

Visualize a muscle pumping a weight. When the muscle becomes exhausted, the weight cannot be pumped or picked up no matter how hard the person tries. If the muscle is rested and re-energized, the weight can again be pumped. The pancreas is similar. Years or decades of chronic insulin overproduction will cause exhaustion. "Resting" the pancreas with diet and improving muscle cell sensitivity to insulin via exercise can restore the pancreas to proper function without medication.

The Amino Solution offers a structure for you to get control of your blood glucose levels and maintain that control over a lifetime of diabetes treatment.

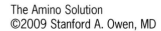

The Amino Solution
©2009 Stanford A. Owen, MD

What Role Might Cytokine Imbalance Play?

Cytokines have been discovered that promote cell "resistance" to insulin (called resistin). Other cytokines directly enhance cell sensitivity to insulin. Further malfunction occurs from cytokines that interfere with the production of or action of the "resistance" or sensitizing cytokines. Whatever the final mechanisms turn out to be, diet and exercise are shown to "balance" these cytokines, helping the body "fix" the metabolism "errors" common in diabetes.

What Results Could I Expect with MNT?

MNT is the primary treatment for Type 2 diabetes mellitus (T2DM), especially therapy that limits the amount of carbohydrates (especially sugars) that you eat or drink. Medication should be added only after trying a glucose-control diet and having that diet fail to produce significant changes in blood sugar. Many people with diabetes, experience something called "diabetic neuropathy," which is nerve damage, frequently described as burning in the feet or legs. These symptoms typically improve, especially if present for only a few years. Other conditions related to diabetes usually improve with MNT as well, including: hypertension, edema (swelling), elevated cholesterol / triglycerides, sleep disorders, fatigue, and depression. Study each applicable disease section, and complete the Disease / Symptom Questionnaires to track exactly how MNT helps with diabetes-related symptoms.

In our clinic, 90 percent of diabetic patients gain control of their diabetes if they precisely follow the 14-day Plan. By restarting Food Phase 1 each time you "go off" the plan, you can regain and maintain glucose control.

Chapter 9: MNT as First-Line Treatment

How Can I Measure Symptom Change on the Plan?

You need to be clear about whether or not you have Type 2/adult onset diabetes mellitus. If monitoring blood sugar with a home test kit (available at pharmacies), record daily glucose readings until they are normal and stay normal (FPG level at less than 126 mg/dl). If you take medications for diabetes, your physician should closely supervise your treatment throughout the MNT Plan.

With your doctor, complete the symptom score sheet below based on the lab tests your doctor takes at each visit.

WHAT DO I NEED TO DO?

1. Monitor daily blood glucose with a home testing kit. Note the change in daily measures during each Food Phase.

2. Have your doctor complete the lab test portions of the Disease/Symptom Questionnaire below before you begin MNT and every 12 weeks thereafter. Discuss what interim measures you should take and whether or not you should use home test kits available at your pharmacy for measuring glucose and hemoglobin A1C between visits.

3. Record any symptoms you have related to circulatory problems associated with diabetes.

4. Indicate how many medications you currently take for diabetes.

5. Review the results with your doctor during each visit. Talk about how you're feeling and whether or not you might need to alter the type or dose of medications you currently take for your diabetes.

DIABETES (TYPE 2) DISEASE/SYMPTOM QUESTIONNAIRE

INITIAL FASTING BLOOD SUGAR* ____ 12-WEEK FASTING BLOOD SUGAR ____	INITIAL HEMOGLOBIN A1C* ____ 12-WEEK HEMOGLOBIN A1C ____
NEUROPATHY PRESENT BURNING LEGS/FEET YES____ NO____ RESTLESS LEGS YES____ NO____ NUMBNESS YES____ NO____	**NEUROPATHY AT 12 WEEKS** BURNING LEGS/FEET YES____ NO____ RESTLESS LEGS YES____ NO____ NUMBNESS YES____ NO____

* Hemoglobin A1C kits and home glucose kits are available at all pharmacies.

Number of Diabetic Medications Used _____(e.g., glyburide + metformin = 2)

* WARNING: NEVER DISCONTINUE A PHYSICIAN-PRESCRIBED MEDICATION WITHOUT CONSULTING WITH YOUR DOCTOR

The most common types of chronic headache — migraine, muscle tension, and pseudotumor — all respond to the MNT Plan for different reasons and at different rates.

HEADACHE (FROM MIGRAINE, MUSCLE TENSION, AND "PSEUDOTUMOR")

What is Headache?

Headache is a common symptom that may result from a number of different problems or illnesses. Headaches are classified as either "primary" or "secondary." Primary headaches are those that occur without appearing to be caused by another illness, such as tension headaches or migraines. Secondary headaches can result from a number of conditions. These may range from life threatening brain tumors, strokes, and meningitis to less serious problems, such as caffeine or pain medication withdrawals.

What Causes Migraine, Muscle Tension, and Pseudotumor-related Headaches?

Migraine is a throbbing headache usually originating in the front or side of the head. Its cause is really not known; however, a number of "triggers" have been identified, such as stress, sleep disturbances, hormones, bright or flickering lights, certain odors, cigarette smoke, alcohol, aged cheeses, chocolate, monosodium glutamate, nitrites, aspartame, and caffeine.

Migraine is often commonly mistaken for "sinus" headache, since migraine often causes congestion. If the throbbing of the headache is sensitive to light or sound OR gets worse when bending or stooping, it is probably migraine.

Pseudotumor cerebri is a condition due to excess spinal fluid pressure; it is most common in people who gain weight and become obese, especially women. The cause is unknown.

Muscle tension headaches often appear to be related to posture problems that occur in those with large abdomens or breasts and improve with treatment for the neck muscles involved. Muscle tension or traction headaches from excess weight may take longer to resolve and relate to total weight loss.

☞ Chapter 9: MNT as First-Line Treatment ☜

What Role Might Cytokine Imbalance Play?

Migraine is due to swelling and inflammation of brain blood vessels. This swelling and inflammation cause irritation of brain nerve fibers which then convey pain across the head and face. The swelling and inflammation are mediated by proteins in the cytokine class. As in other illness, genetic factors play a role. It is possible the inflammatory and swelling related cytokines generated from fat cells, liver, and intestine contribute to these genetic migraine triggers in obesity.

Why **pseudotumor** responds to MNT is also unknown. Hormones and cytokine proteins control spinal fluid regulation in the brain. Cytokines from fat tissue may influence formation or removal of spinal fluid. Only a spinal puncture can diagnose pseudotumor. If headache responds to the PrescriptFit™ MNT Plan, pseudotumor should be considered likely, even without a spinal puncture.

Since pseudotumor predominately affects women, hormones obviously play a role. Exactly how fat-produced cytokines and hormones interplay to prevent removal of spinal fluid is unknown. However, it is likely that cytokines mediate the process. Why? Because headache improves and pressure measures from spinal puncture register decreases in days or weeks after starting the Amino Solution Plan, long before substantial weight loss occurs.

Muscle tension headache will only improve at the rate that the mechanical strain that causes it improves. Weight loss and decreased inflammation will help alleviate mechanical strain sooner. Headaches that improve rapidly on the Plan are probably due to another cause.

Because migraine is 500 percent more common in obesity (although the reason is unknown), MNT is considered a first-line treatment.

MNT is the recommended first-line treatment of pseudotumor to decrease spinal fluid pressure.

The Amino Solution
©2009 Stanford A. Owen, MD

The diet control and design of the Amino Solution Plan allows a more objective way to evaluate the role of diet and obesity on headache.

What Results Could I Expect with MNT?

Clinical experience with MNT and headache varies with the cause. **Pseudotumor** responds within days or weeks but requires a spinal puncture for confirmation. **Migraine** may respond quickly; however, it has many triggers and a naturally variable course. Therefore, long-term response can be gauged only by recording headache scores on the Disease/Symptom Questionnaire over time (e.g., monthly for at least a year). **Muscle tension headache** should respond based on total weight loss.

How Can I Measure Symptom Change on the Plan?

First, you need to be clear about what may be causing your headaches. If your headache is caused by another medical condition or situation (e.g., caffeine withdrawal), work with your doctor to identify the source and plan appropriate treatment. Next, you want to measure how severe each symptom is for you. This will give you a "baseline" to compare with future measurements.

Some people suffer with all three types of headache. Note when and how much your headache improves as well as whether or not headaches return during a particular Food Phase. If this happens, go back to the previous Food Phase and note what happens. If you can't identify a specific Food Phase that relates to the headache returning, start Phase 1 again and proceed forward until you identify a pattern.

Most importantly, you (and your doctor) need a way to measure progress over time. Talk with your doctor at each regular visit about your symptoms and how they might change using the Plan.

As with any medical condition, treatment traditionally means taking medications to reduce symptoms. A number of prescription and over-the-counter medications help alleviate headache pain and, in the case of migraine, provide some prevention. With this Plan, you may find that as symptoms lessen, you need less medication. If you are taking prescription medicines, talk to your doctor about when and how to cut down on what you take BEFORE you make any changes.

≈ Chapter 9: MNT as First-Line Treatment ≈

WHAT DO I NEED TO DO?

1. Check each symptom you are currently experiencing in the Disease/ Symptom Questionnaire below.
2. Grade the level of discomfort you have on a scale from 0–10 (with "0" being no symptom at all to a "10" being severe discomfort) as well as how often you need medication for the pain.
3. Be sure to check the symptoms and grade your level of discomfort AGAIN at the end of each Food Phase or every four weeks.
4. Total the number of medications you currently take for headache, and check the names of any you recognize. Be sure to re-record this information at the end of each Food Phase or every four weeks.
5. Take the results with you to your next doctor's appointment. Talk about how you're feeling and whether or not you still need any prescription medications for headache.

HEADACHE DISEASE/SYMPTOM QUESTIONNAIRE

Headache Symptoms	Level of Discomfort
FREQUENCY	None Constant/Daily **1 2 3 4 5 6 7 8 9 10**
SEVERITY (AVERAGE)	Mild Severe **1 2 3 4 5 6 7 8 9 10**
MEDICATION REQUIRED	Never Always **1 2 3 4 5 6 7 8 9 10**

Headache Medications Used:
Check medications used on a daily basis and total (e.g., aspirin + Tylenol = 2)

MEDICATIONS (CHECK ALL BELOW THAT APPLY. TOTAL MEDICATIONS USED = _____)

- ❏ Aspirin
- ❏ Acetaminophen (Tylenol®)
- ❏ NSAIDS (ibuprofen, naproxen, Vioxx®, Celebrex®, Bextra®, other)
- ❏ Tryptan (Imitrex®, Relpax®, Maxalt®, Zomig®, other)
- ❏ Anti-seizure (Depakote®, Topamax®, Zonegran®, Neurontin®, Gabatril®, Tegretol®, other)
- ❏ Opiates (propoxephene, hydrocodone, meperidine) — Lorcet®, Vicodan®, Oxycontin®, etc.
- ❏ Injectable medication at hospital or clinic

* WARNING: NEVER DISCONTINUE A PHYSICIAN-PRESCRIBED MEDICATION WITHOUT CONSULTING WITH YOUR DOCTOR

The Amino Solution
©2009 Stanford A. Owen, MD

HYPERLIPIDEMIA (ELEVATED CHOLESTEROL AND/OR TRIGLYCERIDES)

What is Hyperlipidemia?

The seven- and 14-day Food Phases should be used when treating cholesterol or triglycerides with the MNT Plan.

Hyperlipidemia is literally the presence of too much fat in the bloodstream. With this condition, you will have elevated cholesterol counts (LDL, HDL, and total cholesterol) and/or triglycerides. Excess levels of these fats speed up the process of hardening of the arteries, which reduces blood flow and can cause heart attack or stroke.

Lowering cholesterol and triglyceride levels decreases this risk. Although some experts believe that current guidelines are not conservative enough, physicians recommend that, to minimize your risk of heart disease, your desirable lipid levels should be:

- LDL less than 130 mg/dL (ideal less than 70)
- HDL greater than 40 mg/dL (men) or 50 mg/dL (women)
- Total cholesterol less than 200 mg/dL (ideal less than 150)
- Triglycerides less than 150 mg/dL

Medications are often required to achieve these levels; however, therapeutic lifestyle changes (TLC), including healthy diet and exercise choices, are considered the first line of treatment.

Hyperlipidemia is the single greatest risk factor for heart disease, although many individuals with "normal" cholesterol levels can develop blockage.

Elevated cholesterol levels do not absolutely predict blockage. Imaging technology may help measure degree of artery blockage. Carotid artery ultrasound and coronary artery calcium deposits can be measured. Coronary calcium scoring is more expensive, and it requires a CT scan.

The Amino Solution
©2009 Stanford A. Owen, MD

⌘ Chapter 9: MNT as First-Line Treatment ⌘

What Causes Hyperlipidemia?

There are two types of hyperlipidemia:

- **The type that runs in families.** If a close relative had early heart disease (father or brother affected before age 55, mother or sister affected before age 65), you also have an increased risk.

- **The type caused by lifestyle habits or treatable medical conditions.** Lifestyle-related causes include obesity, being sedentary, and smoking. Medical conditions that cause hyperlipidemia include diabetes, kidney disease, pregnancy, and having an underactive thyroid gland.

Age can contribute to risk as well — men over 45 and women over 55 are more likely to develop hyperlipidemia.

What Role Might Cytokine Imbalance Play?

The study of atherosclerosis (hardening of the arteries) is now focused primarily in inflammation of the arteries rather than nutritional overload of the bloodstream with fat (although both are important). Cytokines are the primary mediator of inflammation and the focus of most research now is how to reduce cytokine-induced inflammation damage to the arteries. Inflammation leads to cholesterol deposits within the artery, collagen damage resulting in "hardening" or calcification of the artery, and clotting on the damaged surface of the inflamed artery. Diet plays a role in promoting or reducing the degree of inflammation cytokines produce. The Amino Solution optimizes protection from excess cytokine production.

What Results Could I Expect with MNT?

For most of our patients, Food Phases 1 and 2 are associated with the most profound decreases in cholesterol and triglyceride levels.

The Amino Solution
©2009 Stanford A. Owen, MD

MNT is the first-line treatment recommended for hyperlipidemia by every medical textbook and every professional organization. Test cholesterol levels with a home test kit (available at most pharmacies) after each Food Phase or every four weeks of the Plan to evaluate which foods affect cholesterol levels and by how much.

.

Cholesterol blockage of arteries is the most common cause of death and disability — by far. Age, genetic predisposition, diet, obesity, and cigarette smoking significantly increase your risk of cholesterol blockage.

Consider a Carotid Artery Ultrasound or Coronary Calcium CT exam every 1–2 years to measure the actual disease plaque or blockage.

You may see rises in cholesterol levels with some Food Phases that involve some saturated fats, such as those that allow poultry, eggs, pork, beef, dairy, or baked goods. Nuts may actually lower cholesterol levels.

Proving you can control cholesterol with diet, then demonstrating which foods elevate cholesterol, makes infinitely more sense than initially taking a cholesterol-lowering medication. Even if medication is required, diet management is still very important. The learning curve provided by the MNT Plan can be invaluable in deciding if a particular food should be avoided or medication required.

How Can I Measure Lipid Change on the Plan?

First, talk to your doctor about your cholesterol and triglyceride levels as well as your risk level, in general, for heart disease. Have your doctor share with you what your last "lipids screening" results were. This will give you a "baseline" to compare with future measurements. Next, purchase a cholesterol testing kit at a local pharmacy (available without a prescription). Test your cholesterol levels every four weeks if using the recommended 7- or 14-day Plans.

Most importantly, you (and your doctor) need a way to measure progress over time. Talk with your doctor at each regular visit about your symptoms and how they might change using the PrescriptFit™ Plan. Share your test results with your doctor.

As with any medical condition, treatment may mean that you are taking medications to reduce your cholesterol. With MNT, you may find that as symptoms lessen, you need less medication.

Chapter 9: MNT as First-Line Treatment

If taking prescription medicines, talk to you doctor about when and how to cut down on what you take BEFORE you make any changes.

WHAT DO I NEED TO DO?

1. Have the doctor take baseline measurements indicated on the Disease/Symptom Questionnaire below.
2. Purchase a home cholesterol testing kit, and record your results at the end of each Food Phase and 12 weeks after beginning the PrescriptFit™ Plan.
3. Note how each food phase impacts your test results; use this knowledge to determine which food groups might best be avoided.
4. Review the results with your doctor — talk about how you're feeling and whether or not you still need any prescription medications for hyperlipidemia.

HYPERLIPIDEMIA DISEASE/SYMPTOM QUESTIONNAIRE

Food Phase	Total Cholesterol	LDL	HDL	Triglycerides
Baseline Levels				
FOOD PHASE 1				
FOOD PHASE 2				
FOOD PHASE 3				
FOOD PHASE 4				
FOOD PHASE 5				
FOOD PHASE 6				
FOOD PHASE 7				
FOOD PHASE 8				
FOOD PHASE 9				
FOOD PHASE 10				
FOOD PHASE 11				
FOOD PHASE 12				
FOOD PHASE 13				
MAINTENANCE				

* WARNING: NEVER DISCONTINUE A PHYSICIAN-PRESCRIBED MEDICATION WITHOUT CONSULTING WITH YOUR DOCTOR

The Amino Solution
©2009 Stanford A. Owen, MD

HYPERTENSION
(HIGH BLOOD PRESSURE)

What is Hypertension?

Expert guidelines on what actually constitutes "high" blood pressure are when the systolic measurement is above 130 and the diastolic rate is above 85, expressed as 130/85. For those with diabetes or metabolic syndrome (IRS), the goal should be 130/80.

Hypertension or high blood pressure is a condition that signals an overworking heart. Blood pressure is the result of the heart pumping blood into the arteries and the arterial blood vessels exerting resistance to the blood flow from the heart. When either of these forces — diastolic blood pressure (when the heart is resting) or systolic blood pressure (when the heart is beating) is elevated, the heart and arteries have to work under a greater strain. This can cause heart attack, stroke, kidney failure, eye disease, and atherosclerosis (hardening of the arteries). Without treatment, the heart has to work even harder to meet the blood supply needs of the body's organs and tissues, eventually resulting in cardiac disease.

What Causes Hypertension?

There are numerous "primary" factors that can cause hypertension, including obesity, overuse of alcohol, high salt diets, aging, lack of exercise, stress, low potassium, magnesium and calcium intake, and resistance to insulin. Less common is secondary high blood pressure, which occurs as a result of a medication of some other disease (e.g., tumor).

What Role Might Cytokines Play?

For hypertension associated with being overweight or obese, MNT is the first line of treatment because of the direct link between cytokine imbalance and weight loss. Cytokines affect salt and water retention, blood vessel spasm, clotting, and cause direct damage to the collagen structure of blood vessels.

Chapter 9: MNT as First-Line Treatment

Each of these factors alone can contribute to hypertension. All of these factors work together to accelerate hypertension. MNT affects all cytokine components. Therefore, patients with hypertension lose fluid, relax blood vessels, lessen the risk of blood clots, and decrease damage to collagen. MNT is, therefore, a primary treatment of hypertension.

What Results Could I Expect with MNT?

Based on clinical experience for the past decade, the PrescriptFit™ MNT Plan helps patients reduce their need for antihypertensive medication. Because response is typically quite rapid, usually in Food Phase 1 and 2, you must keep in close contact with your physician to avoid medication impacts when the symptoms they treat no longer persist. Close vigilance is required to avoid hypotension (low blood pressure), especially in those using diuretics (fluid-reducing medications), or vasodilators (calcium blockers, alpha blockers).

Talk to your doctor about controlling your hypertension using MNT. Even if medication is initially required to control high blood pressure, MNT may be all you need to later discontinue or decrease the medication you take.

Start out on either the one- or two-week per Food Phase plan, especially if you taking high blood pressure medication. By adding each Food Phase at these intervals, you are more likely to identify particular food groups that contribute to hypertension.

Physician supervision is mandatory, especially in the early Food Phases of the MNT Plan.

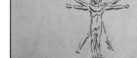

How Can I Measure Symptom Change on the Plan?

Pay special attention to your blood pressure during Food Phase 3 (adding poultry with saturated fat and salt used for taste) and Food Phase 6 (especially for salted nuts). You may need to cook your poultry differently and look for unsalted nuts.

First, you need to be clear about what may be causing your hypertension, especially if it is a secondary problem caused by another medical illness. Talk with your doctor about the cause of your hypertension, possible medication therapy, and what effects MNT may have on that treatment.

Next, you want to take your blood pressure daily. Purchase a home blood pressure monitor and use it at the same time every day, preferably upon waking. This will give you a "baseline" to track improvement or change over time.

Most importantly, you need to work closely with your doctor to balance medications with symptom reduction. Do NOT discontinue or change the way you take prescription medications without consulting with your doctor.

Chapter 9: MNT as First-Line Treatment

WHAT DO I NEED TO DO?

1. Find out if your hypertension results from weight or other diet/lifestyle-related causes.
2. Record your blood pressure at the end of each Food Phase and during the maintenance period after the last Phase (minimum of every 12 weeks).
3. Share the results you've recorded with your doctor. Talk about how you're feeling and whether or not you still need any prescription medications for hypertension.

HYPERTENSION DISEASE/SYMPTOM QUESTIONNAIRE

Food Phase	Systolic Blood Pressure (Average)	Diastolic Blood Pressure (Average)
Baseline Levels		
FOOD PHASE 1		
FOOD PHASE 2		
FOOD PHASE 3		
FOOD PHASE 4		
FOOD PHASE 5		
FOOD PHASE 6		
FOOD PHASE 7		
FOOD PHASE 8		
FOOD PHASE 9		
FOOD PHASE 10		
FOOD PHASE 11		
FOOD PHASE 12		
FOOD PHASE 13		
MAINTENANCE		

* WARNING: NEVER DISCONTINUE A PHYSICIAN-PRESCRIBED MEDICATION WITHOUT CONSULTING WITH YOUR DOCTOR

METABOLIC SYNDROME (INSULIN RESISTANT SYNDROME OR IRS)

What is Insulin/Insulin Resistance?

The PrescriptFit™ MNT Plan is an effective, safe, and rational way to improve insulin resistance. The Plan is first line treatment of IRS.

Insulin is a hormone manufactured in the pancreas and released into the bloodstream when you consume carbohydrates, fats, and protein. Insulin regulates how your body metabolizes carbohydrate, fat, and protein by allowing these nutrients into your cells. The amount of insulin released is finely controlled by a feedback messaging system that relays how quickly and effectively nutrients enter individual cells (especially in the liver and muscle).

If the receptor at the cell surface no longer "allows" insulin to "land" on the cell, excess insulin accumulates in the bloodstream. Despite this overabundance of insulin in the bloodstream, the pancreas "thinks" that your body needs more insulin because the relay system isn't working properly and produces and secretes even more. This "resistance" to the action of insulin is known as the insulin resistant syndrome (or IRS).

Other terms related to IRS include "prediabetes" and "metabolic syndrome"; however, these terms mean slightly different things.

> **Prediabetes** is defined as a time period (perhaps lasting years or decades) prior to a diagnosis of diabetes when insulin metabolism is unhealthy. After years or decades of overwork, the pancreas becomes "exhausted" from the excess insulin production and fails. The result is Type 2 diabetes mellitus (thus giving rise to the term, "prediabetes").

> **Metabolic syndrome** is defined as a group of conditions (i.e., type 2 diabetes, obesity, high blood pressure, and cholesterol problems) that place people at high risk for coronary artery disease. All of the conditions in this group are related to one having excess insulin in his/her bloodstream, which causes defects, especially to adipose tissue and muscle.

Long before obvious diabetes develops, elevated insulin levels in the bloodstream can lead to abnormal metabolism, causing a number of different medical conditions — hypertension (high blood pressure), hyperlipidemia (elevated cholesterol and triglycerides), fatty liver (steatosis), sleep disorders, infertility, and depression. Although IRS can be defined as a cluster of abnormalities (e.g., obesity, hypertension, etc.) associated with insulin resistance and over-secretion of insulin by the pancreas, a cause-and-effect relationship between insulin resistance and the development of these diseases has yet to be conclusively demonstrated.

What determines if you have IRS?

Physicians determine if patients might have IRS by looking for any three of the following:

> **Large waist size:** Does your waist measure more than 35 inches (females) or more than 40" (males)?

> **Blood pressure:** Is your blood pressure greater than 130 systolic/85 diastolic?

> **Fasting blood sugar (FPG):** Do the results of the blood sugar test your doctor runs indicate a blood sugar rate higher than 110?

Additional IRS warning signs include:

- Thick neck
- Skin tags around the neck, arm pit, groin, and face
- Darkening and thickening of the skin of the neck, arm pit, groin, knuckles, elbows, knees, and feet
- Elevated blood insulin levels

> **Fasting triglycerides:** Do the results of a lipid screening indicate that blood levels of triglycerides are greater than 150?

> **HDL cholesterol:** Is your HDL cholesterol at an unhealthy level — less than 40 (for men) or 50 (for women)?

What Role Might Cytokine Imbalance Play?

A cytokine manufactured by fat tissue, called adiponectin, is the primary factor preventing insulin resistance. Decreasing adiponectin levels are associated with increasing insulin levels and diminished insulin function. Diets high in calories, saturated or trans fats, and simple carbohydrate lower adiponectin levels, causing insulin resistance.

Another cytokine manufactured by fat tissue, resistin, causes lower adiponectin levels. Resistin also inhibits the function of insulin on cell surfaces. Elevated resistin secretion is seen in diets high in calories, saturated or trans fats, and simple carbohydrate.

Many fat- and liver-produced cytokines affect adiponectin and resistin levels. Understanding the intricacies of cytokine balance with nutrition is in the earliest phases.

Because having excess adipose (fat) tissue negatively affects how your body regulates insulin production and metabolism, losing weight on a safe, easy-to-follow plan like MNT can't help but ensure success reducing IRS symptoms. Additionally, the overproduction of cytokines due to excess adipose tissue will likely be reduced by the action of the branched-chain amino acids in PrescriptFit™ shakes and soups.

Chapter 9: MNT as First-Line Treatment

What Results Could I Expect with MNT?

Based on our clinical experience, insulin resistance gets better in days to weeks in patients using the PrescriptFit™ MNT Plan. Although the mechanism for how this occurs is unclear, the result is improved sugar metabolism, lower cholesterol, and lower blood pressure.

How Can I Measure Symptom Change on the Plan?

Note that some measurements associated with monitoring IRS must be done by your doctor or in a health care setting, especially tests for cholesterol and blood sugar levels in your bloodstream. Of course, you can monitor your waist size, weight, and blood pressure at home.

First, have your doctor share with you what measurements indicate that you have IRS from the Disease/Symptom Questionnaire on the next page. This will give you a "baseline" to compare with future measurements.

Most importantly, you (and your doctor) need a way to measure progress over time. Talk with your doctor at each regular visit about your symptoms and how they might change using the PrescriptFit™ Plan. Be sure to have your doctor take the same measurements after 12 weeks on the MNT Plan as you took at the beginning.

As with any medical condition, treatment may mean that you are taking medications to reduce symptoms associated with IRS (e.g., hypertension). With PrescriptFit™, you may find that as your symptoms lessen, you will need to take less medication OR perhaps discontinue your medications entirely. If you are taking prescription medicines, talk to you doctor about when and how to cut down on what you take BEFORE you make any changes.

WHAT DO I NEED TO DO?

1. See your physician to determine if you are insulin resistant. Have the doctor take baseline measurements indicated on the Disease/Symptom Questionnaire below.

2. Be sure to have your physician measure the same indicators 12 weeks after beginning the MNT Plan.

3. Review the results with your doctor — talk about how you're feeling and whether or not you still need any prescription medications for conditions related to IRS.

IRS DISEASE/SYMPTOM QUESTIONNAIRE

Disease Measures	Baseline	End of Phase 12*
BLOOD PRESSURE (SYSTOLIC/DIASTOLIC)	_____/_____	_____/_____
FASTING PLASMA GLUCOSE	_____mg/dL	_____mg/dL
FASTING TRIGLYCERIDES	_____mg/dL	_____mg/dL
WAIST CIRCUMFERENCE	_____inches	_____inches
C-PEPTIDE INSULIN LEVEL	_____mg/dL	_____mg/dL
SKIN TAGS (YES OR NO)	_____	_____
ACANTHOSIS ** **(YES OR NO)**	_____	_____

* Those with IRS may not be able to do Food Phase 13 due to carbohydrate restrictions.

** Dark discoloration and thickened skin of neck, axilla, elbows, knuckles, feet

* WARNING: NEVER DISCONTINUE A PHYSICIAN-PRESCRIBED MEDICATION WITHOUT CONSULTING WITH YOUR DOCTOR

Chapter 9: MNT as First-Line Treatment

IRRITABLE BOWEL SYNDROME (IBS)

What is Irritable Bowel Syndrome (IBS)?

IBS is one of the more common maladies affecting adults. As the name implies, IBS feels like the bowel is irritable or "angry." People with IBS experience cramps, diarrhea, feelings of constipation, and generalized abdominal pain usually experienced in the lower abdomen. "Bloating" is a common complaint, especially after meals.

What Causes IBS?

There may be several causes for IBS. One of the more common is the inability to digest certain sugars, which ferment because of the bacteria present in the digestive tract into the gases methane, butane, and formate. These gases are irritating to the gut, produce abnormal motility, and are quite smelly (they are components of "swamp gas" and are quite flammable). These gases have also been associated with generalized muscle pain (similar to fibromyalgia).

You should see your doctor about any ongoing abdominal pain. You will probably need to have some diagnostic tests performed to rule out serious gut disease: peptic ulcers, cancer, ulcerative colitis, or Crohn's Disease (ileitis).

What Role Might Cytokine Imbalance Play?

Cytokines probably play a minimal role in IBS, although the relationship to diet and gut hormone production is being studied. We know that specific gut hormones [e.g., cholecystokinin (CCK), ghrelin, motilin, gastrin] are released in different amounts and patterns depending on meal consistency. We also know that inflammatory cytokines are

All adults over 50 should have a baseline colonoscopy (and follow up every 10 years thereafter) to detect colon cancer in early stages, while still curable. Colonoscopy should be performed earlier if one has a strong family history of colon cancer, if bleeding has occurred, or if symptoms do not improve.

If you suspect that you have IBS, you should probably use the 7-day MNT Plan, adding Food Phases every week. This allows enough time to clearly distinguish what foods are "offenders" to IBS.

While the plan may be boring for a couple of weeks, most patients with troublesome IBS find the boredom worth the effort.

Because IBS is not a harmful condition, experimenting with offending foods will cause no harm; it will only help make changes that eliminate irritating symptoms.

related to an abnormal amount or pattern of gut hormone release. However, no consistent cause-effect relationship has yet been established.

What Results Could I Expect with MNT?

This Plan is an ideal way to test for and improve symptoms of IBS. Many patients improve or resolve using PrescriptFit™ strategies without the need for costly tests or medication. In our clinical experience, most patients report rapid results, often noting improvements the first week.

Food Phase 1 requires use of PrescriptFit™ lactose-free products only (no other food). You should take at least eight doses per day along with a complete multivitamin. You may consume as many as 20 doses per day, if needed, to feel satisfied.

If you are taking medication, especially for high blood pressure, diabetes, acid reflux, or cardiac disease, your physician will need to carefully monitor your condition throughout the Plan.

Food Phases likely to cause symptom recurrence are vegetables, fruit, dairy products, and starchy foods. Sugars found in milk, fruit, beans (legumes), and wheat "ferment" in the gut to form methane, butane, and formate. By adding each food group sequentially, you can identify and then avoid the offending foods. Use this four-step, "trial-and-error" approach to "weed out" the foods that make you feel bad:

1. If symptoms increase during a particular Food Phase, simply skip that phase.

2. Add Phases and note symptoms.

3. If symptoms occur in subsequent Food Phases, skip those phases as well until all 13 Food Phases are complete.

Chapter 9: MNT as First-Line Treatment

4. Sequentially add previously offensive Food Phases and note results.

How Can I Measure Symptom Change on the PrescriptFit™ Plan?

First, you need to be clear about what symptoms of IBS you might have. Next, you want to measure how severe each symptom is for you. This will give you a "baseline" to compare with future measurements. Most importantly, you (and your doctor) need a way to measure progress over time. Talk with your doctor at each regular visit about your symptoms and how they might change using the PrescriptFit™ Plan.

The simplicity of the PrescriptFit™ IBS approach is that one group of foods, like dairy, may be well tolerated, while fruit and wheat (baked goods) may not. What a treat to find the offenders while preserving the delights!

WHAT DO I NEED TO DO?

1. Check each symptom you are currently experiencing in the Disease/Symptom Questionnaire below.
2. Grade the level of discomfort you have on a scale from 0–10 (with "0" being no symptom at all to a "10" being severe discomfort).
3. Be sure to check the symptoms and grade your level of discomfort AGAIN at the end of each Food Phase or every four weeks.
4. Take the results with you to your next doctor's appointment. Talk about how you're feeling and whether or not you still need any prescription medications for IBS.

IBS Disease/Symptom Questionnaire

Symptom Experience	Level of Discomfort
ABDOMINAL PAIN (CRAMPING, BLOATING, ACHING)	None ... Severe 0 1 2 3 4 5 6 7 8 9 10
GAS	None ... Severe 0 1 2 3 4 5 6 7 8 9 10
DIARRHEA	None ... Severe 0 1 2 3 4 5 6 7 8 9 10
CONSTIPATION	None ... Severe 0 1 2 3 4 5 6 7 8 9 10

* WARNING: NEVER DISCONTINUE A PHYSICIAN-PRESCRIBED MEDICATION WITHOUT CONSULTING WITH YOUR DOCTOR

The Amino Solution
©2009 Stanford A. Owen, MD

Snoring may be a key indicator of sleep apnea; it is common with aging and in those with sleep disorders.

Sleep disorders are studied in certified sleep laboratories available in most communities.

SLEEP APNEA / SNORING

What is Sleep Apnea?

Sleep apnea is a sleep disorder that affects some 18 million Americans and can be very serious if not treated. People with this disorder stop breathing for 10 to 30 seconds at a time while they are sleeping, possibly as many as 400 times each night. These periods of not breathing often wake you from deep sleep, seriously reducing the amount of necessary rest you actually get.

Those with sleep apnea typically suffer progressive fatigue, tiredness, malaise, depression, and muscle stiffness. Sleep apnea is associated with increased risk for heart attack and stroke. In addition, this common disorder can lead to disability and death from motor vehicle accidents that occur when the person falls asleep at the wheel from extreme tiredness.

Treatment typically involves use of dental devices, equipment that increases air pressure to increase restful breathing during sleep, and weight loss.

What Causes Sleep Apnea?

"Obstructive" sleep apnea is what nine out of 10 people with sleep apnea have and is caused by something blocking the passage or windpipe (called the trachea) that brings air into your body. That something may be:

> Your tongue, tonsils, or the uvula (the small piece of flesh hanging down in the back of the throat).

> Excessive fatty tissue in the throat; many people with sleep apnea are obese.

> Abnormally relaxed throat muscles, due to poor function of the nerves from the

Chapter 9: MNT as First-Line Treatment

lower brain that control breathing and swallowing. Evidence suggest the poor nerve function is related to abnormal metabolism.

What Role Might Cytokine Imbalance Play?

The exact role that cytokines have on sleep is unknown. Studies show that most sleep apnea patients have excess levels of cytokines associated with inflammation, which attach directly to nerve cells in the brain, including the areas that control breathing and swallowing.

What Results Could I Expect with MNT?

MNT is the first line of treatment recommended in obese or overweight patients with sleep disorders. Patients using the Plan note improvement in fatigue by the end of Food Phases 1 and 2 of the 7- to 14-day Plans.

With MNT, many patients can eventually discontinue annoying and expensive sleep devices. Nutritional diets appear to be far more important than weight loss in treating sleep apnea. In most patients, improvement in fatigue and snoring diminishes long before large weight loss is noted. In fact, patients who undergo gastric bypass operations often can stop using special breathing devices for sleep apnea within weeks — long before they experience significant weight loss.

How Can I Measure Symptom Change on the Plan?

First, you need to be clear about what may be causing your sleep apnea. Although rare, there is a second type of sleep apnea (central sleep apnea) that occurs when the muscles you use to breathe fail for some reason to receive the signal to do so from your brain. You should work with your physician to clearly identify which type of sleep apnea you have and what would be the best treatment approach. Talk with your doctor about the effects that MNT may have on your treatment. Next, you want to measure how severe each of the two, key sleep apnea symptoms are for you. This will give you a "baseline" to compare with future measurements.

Most importantly, you (and your doctor) need a way to measure progress over time. Talk with your doctor at each regular visit about your symptoms and how they might change using the Plan.

WHAT DO I NEED TO DO?

1. Check your level of energy and snoring in the Disease/Symptom Questionnaire below. For snoring, your partner may be more knowledgeable about your symptoms than you are.

2. Grade the level of discomfort you have on a scale from 0–10 (with "0" being normal energy and no snoring, respectively, and "10" being no energy and severe snoring, respectively).

3. Be sure to check the symptoms and grade your level of discomfort AGAIN at the end of each Food Phase or every four weeks.

4. Take the results with you to your next doctor's appointment. Talk about how you're feeling and whether or not you still need conventional treatments for sleep apnea.

SLEEP APNEA DISEASE/SYMPTOM QUESTIONNAIRE

Symptom Experience	Level of Discomfort	
FATIGUE/ENERGY LEVEL	Normal Energy	No Energy
	0 1 2 3 4 5 6 7 8 9 10	
SNORING	None	Severe
	0 1 2 3 4 5 6 7 8 9 10	

* WARNING: NEVER DISCONTINUE A PHYSICIAN-PRESCRIBED MEDICATION WITHOUT CONSULTING WITH YOUR DOCTOR

The Amino Solution
©2009 Stanford A. Owen, MD

STEATOSIS (FATTY LIVER)

What is Steatosis?

Steatosis or "fatty liver" is the most common form of chronic liver disease, replacing alcohol and viral hepatitis as the most common cause of cirrhosis of the liver. Patients with fatty liver and alcoholism or viral hepatitis are much more likely to have liver cell damage and cirrhosis.

What Causes Fatty Liver?

Fatty liver is caused by the accumulation of triglyceride fat deposits within liver cells due to abnormal liver metabolism. Excessive fat in liver cells provokes inflammation and activates the immune system. Simple blood tests can suggest the presence of inflammation caused by these fat deposits but cannot assure the definitive cause.

Because the only way to prove a diagnosis of steatosis is to perform a biopsy of the liver (which carries a risk of bleeding), many physicians make the diagnosis by exclusion. That is, for those who have NEITHER a history of alcoholism nor lab results indicating a viral/immune liver disease, there is a 90 percent chance that your symptoms indicate a fatty liver — odds reasonable enough to avoid biopsy.

If your doctor finds that your lab tests do not improve or normalize when you carefully follow the Plan, a biopsy may be required.

What Role Might Cytokine Imbalance Play?

Most patients with fatty liver are overweight. Patients with fatty liver have elevated levels of inflammation cytokines (CRP, IL-6, TNF). Patients with fatty liver often have diabetes or pre-diabetes (IRS), conditions also associated with abnormal cytokine production. Studies suggest the fat accumulation and the inflammation of the liver cell are related but independent abnormalities. Common cytokines may play a role in both, and nutrition may be the common mediator.

People with fatty liver tend to be more likely to suffer with metabolic syndrome (insulin resistant syndrome) and eventually become diabetic. They have a higher rate of hypertension and sleep apnea as well as elevated cholesterol and triglyceride levels.

What Results Could I Expect with MNT?

MNT is the first line of treatment for fatty liver, especially because of the Plan's ability to help you reduce your triglyceride levels. Patients using the Plan improve laboratory tests of fatty liver usually by the end of Food Phase 8 of the 7-day or Food Phase 4 of the 14-day Plan. Your physician should perform liver function tests (SGOT, SGPT, and alkaline phosphatase blood tests) every 12 weeks when using the Plan.

How Can I Measure Symptom Change on the Plan?

Improvement in fatty liver enzyme results must be measured by your physician. Share the Disease/Symptom Questionnaire below with your physician; measurement should be considered every 12 weeks until your lab results indicate that the maximum response has been achieved.

STEATOSIS (FATTY LIVER) DISEASE/SYMPTOM QUESTIONNAIRE	
INITIAL LAB VALUES	**12-WEEK LAB VALUES**
SGOT _____	**SGOT** _____
SGPT _____	**SGPT** _____
ALKALINE PHOSPHATASE _____	**ALKALINE PHOSPHATASE** _____

* WARNING: NEVER DISCONTINUE A PHYSICIAN-PRESCRIBED MEDICATION WITHOUT CONSULTING WITH YOUR DOCTOR

CHAPTER 10: ENHANCING WELLNESS WITH MNT

The Plan is designed to help you discover for yourself how to craft your most successful lifestyle by letting you learn what works and what doesn't at each step of nutrition change. You will probably experience some remission *(absence or significant reduction of troublesome symptoms)* as well as relapse *(a return to illness)*. Because PrescriptFit™ measures outcome, you quickly learn how and where to adjust your plan away from danger and toward health.

MNT can be used as to assist treatment for a number of illnesses and chronic conditions, such as:

> Angina Pectoris

> Arthritis (Inflammatory Type)

> Asthma / Allergies

> Back Pain

> Congestive Heart Failure

> Depression

> Dyspnea (Breathlessness)

> Edema (Swelling)

> Fatigue

> Fibromyalgia

> Infertility

> Insomnia

> Joint Pain (Degenerative Type)

> Sexual Dysfunction

The Amino Solution
©2009 Stanford A. Owen, MD

Angina Pectoris
(Chest Pain; Heart Pain; Chest Pressure; Chest Heaviness)

What is Angina Pectoris?

Half of all heart attack victims die prior to reaching medical care; yet most experienced warning symptoms.

Angina is described as pain, pressure, crushing, pressing, heavy, or breathless discomfort in the chest. Angina may radiate to the back, neck, or down the arms. It may be mild to severe.

Angina may be precipitated by exertion, emotion, food, smoking, sleeplessness, altitude, and other factors that alter the tone of small blood vessels. It is often worse in the morning.

Any angina symptoms (not previously diagnosed by a physician) warrant immediate attention.

Angina can be both disabling and frightening. Usually present prior to a heart attack, angina is often ignored as "indigestion" or associated with fatigue and exhaustion (especially in women).

What Causes Angina Pectoris?

Angina pain originates from the heart, caused by insufficient blood flow through the arteries caused by spasm or cholesterol blockage of the coronary arteries.

What Role Might Cytokine Imbalance Play?

Small blood vessels react to changes in excess calories, sugar, and fat. Improvement in blood vessel function improves using branched-chain amino acids. Cytokines have direct influence on small vessel lining to cause spasm, increase clotting, and damage collagen that keeps the vessel supple and pliable.

What Results Could I Expect with MNT?

Those using the Plan often note immediate and substantial relief of angina, especially in Food Phases 1 and 2. Likewise, patients may experience immediate pain relapse even after a large meal, especially if high in fat and sugar.

The Amino Solution
©2009 Stanford A. Owen, MD

Chapter 10: Enhancing Wellness with MNT

Angina may be very sensitive to amount of food, type of food, and even preparation of food (as with use of fatty condiments). Remain alert to improvement and relapse of symptoms.

How Can I Measure Symptom Change on the Plan?

Angina can be sporadic or predictable. If your experience with angina is predictable, you will find improvement the easiest to measure. For example, you may feel angina every time you walk to the mailbox up the hill and have to rest or take a nitroglycerine tablet to resolve the discomfort. Being able to complete the walk without stopping would be a measurable improvement you could readily see. If your experience with angina is more sporadic, it may take some time to see a trend that indicates less episodes of discomfort.

First, you need to make sure that you see your physician immediately for any symptoms of angina that have not been previously diagnosed. Your doctor will prescribe treatment after determining what course of cardiac care is best for you. You will need to follow that treatment carefully. MNT can support your treatment plan with the combined benefits of branched-chain amino acids and how you monitor changes throughout the Food Phases.

Next, you want to have a measurement of how frequent, severe, and long lasting each episode of angina is for you. This will give you a "baseline" to compare with future measurements.

Most importantly, you (and your doctor) need a way to measure progress over time. Talk with your doctor at each visit about your symptoms and how they might change using the Plan.

Of medications prescribed to reduce symptoms, nitroglycerin is perhaps the best known. However, you should record whether or not you take this medication and if it offers relief during the episodes you measure. Also record the same information for other medications your physician may prescribe for this condition.

WHAT DO I NEED TO DO?

1. Determine how often you experience angina in the Disease/Symptom Questionnaire below.
2. Grade the level of discomfort you have, as well as, the duration of the discomfort on the Questionnaire as indicated.
3. Indicate whether nitroglycerin and/or other medications prescribed relieved the discomfort.
4. Be sure to grade your angina episodes AGAIN at the end of each Food Phase or every four weeks.
5. Take the results with you to your next doctor's appointment. Talk about how you're feeling and whether you still need any prescription medications for angina.
6. If symptoms relapse, return to the previous Phase and progress again. If angina returns with the same Food Phase each time, eliminate the provoking food. When returning to prior Phases, progress through each one more slowly to clearly identify the offending food group.

ANGINA PECTORIS DISEASE/SYMPTOM QUESTIONNAIRE

Angina Discomfort

FREQUENCY	❏ DAILY	❏ <3/DAY	❏ ≥ 3/DAY
INTENSITY (AVERAGE)	❏ MILD	❏ MODERATE	❏ SEVERE
DURATION	❏ ≤ 1 MINUTE	❏ ≤ 5 MINUTES	❏ ≤ 30 MINUTES

Relief from Medications

NITROGLYCERIN	❏ YES ❏ No
OTHER MEDICATION (ANGINA PREVENTION OR TREATMENT)	❏ YES ❏ No

* WARNING: NEVER DISCONTINUE A PHYSICIAN-PRESCRIBED MEDICATION WITHOUT CONSULTING WITH YOUR DOCTOR

The Amino Solution
©2009 Stanford A. Owen, MD

ASTHMA

What is Asthma?

Asthma can be caused by an allergic reaction or triggered by a number of factors not related to allergies. Exercises, exposure to cold air, or heartburn are some non-allergy related triggers. Environmental factors, such as tobacco smoke, pollutants, and stress, as well as biological factors, related to ones internal chemistry, appear to trigger attacks.

What Causes Asthma?

The main contributor to asthma is inflammation within the lungs. This leads to constriction of the airway muscles, stimulation of mucus production, and flooding of the airways with inflammatory cells.

The main contributor to asthma is inflammation within the lungs leading to constriction of the airway muscles, stimulation of mucous production, and flooding of the airways with inflammatory cells.

What Role Might Cytokine Imbalance Play?

Cytokines trigger inflammation that may result in asthma. Branched chain amino acids may improve out of balance cytokines and significantly reduce symptoms. Most new asthma medications directly attack cytokines (called leukotrienes). Therefore, logic dictates a trial of MNT to measure asthma improvement.

The incidence of asthma is increased markedly in the obese (both children and adults). The epidemic increase of asthma in children that has occurred in the last two decades may be, in part, related to the epidemic of childhood obesity.

The beauty of the Food Phase Plan is your ability to carefully add in each food group and isolate exactly which foods might trigger asthma attacks.

Note that some measurements associated with monitoring asthma must be done by your doctor or in a health care setting, especially measurements of lung flow (referred to as the "Peak Flow" test). Peak Flow "meters" are available at any drugstore and are recommended for asthma patients home use.

What Results Could I Expect with MNT?

Based on clinical data, asthma improves in many patients using the MNT Plan, especially in Food Phases 1 and 2. Additionally, PrescriptFit™ may improve asthma by removing the thousands of different nutrients, bacteria, and chemicals in a normal diet. Food Phases 1 and 2 of the Plan limit exposure to nutrients and particles that might trigger inflammation. As a specific food group is added in, note if asthma worsens. A specific food group may contribute to asthma in one person but not another. Those foods high in fat, sugar, and dairy products should be especially monitored to see if symptoms worsen after eating.

How Can I Measure Symptom Change on the Plan?

First, see your doctor right away for any symptoms of asthma. Have your doctor share with you what measurements indicate that you have asthma and if your asthma might be from an allergy. Next, complete the Disease/Symptom Questionnaire at right for a "baseline" to compare with future measures.

Most importantly, you (and your doctor) need a way to measure progress over time. Talk with your doctor at each regular visit about your symptoms and how they might change using the Plan. Be sure to have your doctor take the same measurements after 12 weeks on the MNT Plan as you had taken at the "baseline" mark.

With PrescriptFit™, you may find that as your symptoms lessen, you will need to take less medication OR perhaps discontinue your medications entirely. If you are taking prescription medicines, talk to you doctor about when and how to cut down on what you take.

⌐ Chapter 10: Enhancing Wellness with MNT ⌐

WHAT DO I NEED TO DO?

1. See your physician to determine if you have asthma and whether an allergy might be related to your symptoms. Have the doctor take a baseline measurement of lung flow and record the results.

2. Rate your level of discomfort/severity as indicated on the Disease/Symptom Questionnaire below on a scale of 0–10, with "0" indicating mild symptoms and "10" indicating the most severe problems. Re-measure asthma symptoms after each Food Phase of the Plan.

3. Record the type of inhaler and frequency of use, as well as, other medications your doctor prescribes on the Questionnaire below.

4. Note how quickly and completely symptoms resolve. When symptoms relapse, note which food phase you are in, return to the one before, and proceed again. Note relapse that occurs at the same phase each time.

5. Have your physician measure lung flow 12 weeks after beginning the Plan.

6. Review results with your doctor; ask how your medication needs may change as your symptoms change.

ASTHMA DISEASE/SYMPTOM QUESTIONNAIRE

Symptom	Level of Discomfort
BREATHLESSNESS	Mild　　　　　　　Moderate　　　　　　Severe 0　1　2　3　4　5　6　7　8　9　10
COUGHING	Infrequent　　　　Frequent　　　　　Constant 0　1　2　3　4　5　6　7　8　9　10
WHEEZING	Occasional　　　　Often　　　　　　Constant 0　1　2　3　4　5　6　7　8　9　10
SPUTUM PRODUCTION	None　　Minimal　　Moderate　　　Constant 0　1　2　3　4　5　6　7　8　9　10
IMPACT ON QUALITY OF LIFE	None　Nuisance　Interferes　Alters　Threatens 0　1　2　3　4　5　6　7　8　9　10

Lung Flow Measure (physician testing): Peak Flow _____liters/minute

INHALERS **FREQUENCY OF USE** **NUMBER USED** (CHECK THOSE USED AND TOTAL) **TOTAL** _____	Daily (puffs/day): ❏1　❏2　❏3　❏4　❏>4 Weekly (days/week): ❏1　❏2　❏3　❏4　❏>4 ❏ ALBUTEROL /SALBUTEROL　❏ STEROID INHALER ❏ COMBINATION INHALERS (COMBIVENT™, ADVAIR™) ❏ ATROVENT　　　　　　　❏ CHROMALYN
ORAL MEDICATIONS:	❏ THEOPHYLLINE　❏ BRETHINE

* WARNING: NEVER DISCONTINUE PRESCRIBED MEDICATION WITHOUT CONSULTING WITH A DOCTOR

The Amino Solution
©2009 Stanford A. Owen, MD

BACK PAIN

What is Back Pain?

Back pain is an ongoing aching, soreness, and/ or strained feeling in the back anywhere from the shoulders to the hips. It occurs in everyone at some point in life. It can result from some acute injury as well as chronic strain from poor posture, excessive weight, or both. Some health conditions, such as kidney infection, can cause severe pain and soreness in the mid portion of the back. You should always consult with your doctor about any unexplained back pain to be sure that you are not suffering from some illness that requires immediate treatment.

What Causes Back Pain?

For chronic back pain that results from ongoing strain due to weight, cause is related to your body's attempts to adjust your form to your changing body shape. As weight increases, abdominal size expands forward, causing stress along the ligaments and muscles connecting the vertebrae and collagen discs; the result — chronic pain.

What Role Might Cytokine Imbalance Play?

There is evidence that cytokines produced by fat cells may lead to direct injury of collagen, weakening the ligaments, tendons, and spinal discs. Fat cells also produce inflaming cytokine proteins that may damage the lining of joints, including the small joints separating each vertebrae that allow you to easily bend, twist, and stretch the spine.

Back pain is present in almost every obese person.

Chapter 10: Enhancing Wellness with MNT

What Results Could I Expect with MNT?

The MNT Plan will reduce the excessive weight and cytokines that contribute to back strain. Based on over a decade of clinical experience, 67 percent of patients who visit our clinic can discontinue medication for back pain within six months after they begin using the MNT Plan combined with physical therapy or rehabilitative exercise. For those taking anti-inflammatory medications for back pain, there's an added bonus of stomach complaints improving — both from the reduced need to take the anti-inflammatory medications AND from eliminating irritating foods using the MNT Food Phase approach to identify those causing digestive problems.

How Can I Measure Symptom Change on the Plan?

First, you need to be clear about what is causing your back pain. If you're overweight, work in a job that requires lifting and other strenuous activities, or have recently strained your back, you should talk to your doctor about the benefits of the MNT Plan as well as physical therapy / rehabilitative exercise. If your back pain has occurred recently without explanation or apparent cause, your doctor will need to determine if there might be a more serious illness causing your discomfort that requires treatment.

Next, you want to have a measurement of how severe your back pain is on a daily basis. This will give you a "baseline" to compare with future measurements.

Most importantly, you (and your doctor) need a way to measure progress over time. Talk with your doctor at each regular visit about your symptoms and how they have changed using the Plan.

As with any medical condition, treatment traditionally means taking medications to reduce symptoms. A number of prescription and over-the-counter medications can be taken to reduce the pain and inflammation in your back. With MNT, you may find that you will need to take less medication OR perhaps discontinue your medications entirely. If you are taking prescription medicines, talk to your doctor about when and how to cut down on what you take BEFORE you make any changes.

WHAT DO I NEED TO DO?

1. Grade the level of daily discomfort you have on a scale from 0–10 (with "0" being mild and "10" being severe discomfort).

2. Be sure to grade your level of discomfort AGAIN at the end of each Food Phase or every four weeks.

3. Record the number of medications you currently take for back pain. Be sure to record how many pain medications you're taking at the end of each Food Phase or every four weeks.

4. Take the results with you to your next doctor's appointment. Talk about how you're feeling and whether you still need medications for back pain.

BACK PAIN DISEASE/SYMPTOM QUESTIONNAIRE

AVERAGE DAILY BACK PAIN	Mild Moderate Severe 0 1 2 3 4 5 6 7 8 9 10
NUMBER OF MEDICATIONS TAKEN DAILY _____ (E.G., ASPIRIN + TYLENOL = 2 MEDICATIONS)	

* WARNING: NEVER DISCONTINUE A PHYSICIAN-PRESCRIBED MEDICATION WITHOUT CONSULTING WITH YOUR DOCTOR

The Amino Solution
©2009 Stanford A. Owen, MD

CONGESTIVE HEART FAILURE (CHF)

What is Congestive Heart Failure (CHF)?

Congestive Heart Failure occurs when the heart can't pump enough blood to supply the body's organs. "Back-pressure" of blood leads to lung congestion, producing breathlessness and shortness of breath. The kidney has more trouble getting rid of sodium and water when blood flow is compromised, which results in swelling (edema) of the legs.

Patients with CHF struggle to breathe when walking, wake up at night breathless, and "give out" easily.

Patients with CHF often demonstrate dramatic improvement using the PrescriptFit™ MNT Plan. MNT should be an integral part of CHF treatment since type and amount of nutrients affect fluid retention.

What Causes CHF?

Age and obesity are the two major causes of CHF. As heart tissue ages, it has more trouble pumping blood with the same efficiency of a "younger" heart. Similarly, the heart must pump substantially harder when one is obese. CHF can also result from heart muscle damage after a heart attack, prolonged uncontrolled high blood pressure, and malfunctioning heart valves. Nutritional deficiency further weakens heart muscle cells.

Cytokines play a dominant role in CHF via fluid balance, excess clotting, repair and renewal of injured heart cells, and small blood vessel malfunction. The dramatic improvement seen in CHF patients (under physician guidance) with MNT may be, in part,

> Patients with CHF should use PrescriptFit™ MNT Plan only under direct and close medical supervision.

due to balancing of cytokine function. Excess fluid is removed, blood vessels relax, clotting diminishes, and heart cells function better. Scarring of the heart lessens.

What Results Could I Expect with MNT?

In our clinic, improvement with MNT has been unrelated to amount of weight loss. Certainly, decreased weight equals decreased stress on the heart. However, the percentage improvement noted typically occurs within the first 12 weeks of starting MNT, usually in the first two weeks — long before meaningful fat loss occurs. Patients who comply with the Amino Solution maintenance strategies following all Food Phases can often diminish fluid medication with physician guidance. **CHF patients should keep in close contact with their doctor during Food Phase 1. Do not regulate medication on your own.**

Use the 14-day Plan to clearly determine which food groups or what quantity of food will cause fluid retention. While difficult to follow, the improvement usually far outweighs the deprivation. Even a 7-day/Phase strategy provides significant improvement in most cases.

How Can I Measure Symptom Change on the Plan?

First, you need to be clear about what might be causing your symptoms of CHF. Visit your doctor to determine if edema or shortness of breath could stem from some other illness. Next, you want to have a measurement of how severe each symptom is for you. This will give you a "baseline" to compare with future measurements.

Patients with CHF can lose 20–50 pounds of fluid in Food Phases 1 and 2, demonstrating the powerful effect of dietary influences on cardiovascular physiology.

Tell your doctor about the review available in the *American Journal of Cardiology Supplement*, April 2004: "The Role of Nutritional Supplements with Essential Amino Acids in Patients with Cardiovascular Disease and Diabetes Mellitus."

Chapter 10: Enhancing Wellness with MNT

Most importantly, you (and your doctor) need a way to measure progress over time. Talk with your doctor at each visit about your symptoms and how they might change using the PrescriptFit™ Plan.

As with any medical condition, treatment traditionally means taking medications to reduce symptoms. With PrescriptFit™, you may find that as your symptoms lessen, you will need to take less medication OR perhaps discontinue your medications entirely.

If you are taking prescription medicines, talk to your doctor about when and how to cut down on what you take BEFORE you make any changes.

WHAT DO I NEED TO DO?

1. Check each symptom you are currently experiencing in the Disease/Symptom Questionnaire below.
2. Grade the level of discomfort you have on a scale from 0–10 (with "0" being no symptom or problem and "10" being severe discomfort or lack of stamina).
3. Be sure to check the symptoms and grade your level of discomfort AGAIN at the end of each Food Phase or every four weeks.
4. Take the results with you to your next doctor's appointment. Talk about how you're feeling and what changes you might be able to make to your prescribed medications for CHF.

CONGESTIVE HEART FAILURE DISEASE/SYMPTOM QUESTIONNAIRE

Symptom Experience	Level of Discomfort	
EDEMA/FLUID RETENTION	None 0 1 2 3 4 5 6 7 8 9 10	Severe
SHORTNESS OF BREATH	None 0 1 2 3 4 5 6 7 8 9 10	Severe
ORTHOPNEA (INABILITY TO BREATHE EASILY WHEN LYING FLAT)	No Problem 0 1 2 3 4 5 6 7 8 9 10	Severe
STAMINA/SENSE OF WELL BEING	Normal 0 1 2 3 4 5 6 7 8 9 10	No Stamina

* WARNING: NEVER DISCONTINUE A PHYSICIAN-PRESCRIBED MEDICATION WITHOUT CONSULTING WITH YOUR DOCTOR

The Amino Solution
©2009 Stanford A. Owen, MD

Depression

What is Depression?

Depression is a chronic psychiatric condition that can be very debilitating or even life threatening. People who are depressed will typically feel sad and hopeless, may have changes in eating and sleeping patterns, and may move and think more slowly than usual. If severe, they may think about or plan suicide. The most common symptoms include being fatigued and unable to get motivated to participate in or enjoy activities that used to be pleasurable (including sex).

What Causes Depression?

We don't know exactly what causes depression; however, experts agree that some people are more prone to depression than others and that certain events or situations can put these people at risk for suffering from the illness. What we do know is that there are chemicals in the brain that impact how we handle stress, and these chemicals appear to be out of balance for those diagnosed with depression.

Many medical conditions and some medications can contribute to symptoms of depression. People with depression often struggle with anxiety or mood swings as well. In addition, poor nutrition may contribute to depression. People who are depressed often either eat too much because it's soothing or eat too little because they have no appetite or energy for eating. Nutritional balance certainly suffers either way.

What Role Might Cytokine Imbalance Play?

Brain chemicals (called neurotransmitters) are intimately influenced by cytokines produced

See your doctor about any depression symptoms lasting more than two weeks; a thorough evaluation by a physician experienced in treating depression is very important for arriving at the right diagnosis and getting optimal therapy.

by fat, liver, and immune tissues. Depression is more common, for instance, in patients who overproduce C-Reactive Protein (or CRP) — common in those with metabolic syndrome, heart disease, and diabetes. Other cytokines called "interleukins" (IL-6, IL-2, and others) are closely tied to depression. The most dramatic example is the adverse side effect experienced by some when taking interferon (related to interleukin). Interferon is used for treating viral hepatitis; the profound depression that results in many cases often requires discontinuing the treatment.

Other cytokine hormones (leptin, ghrelin, cholecystokinin) have dramatic effects on eating behavior, which in turn, may lead to metabolic problems that contribute to depression.

The brain's nerve cells have receptors that are very sensitive to changes in cytokine production, nutrition balance, and external factors. The common receptors known to affect depression (serotonin, dopamine, and norepinephrine) are also intricately tied to energy metabolism. Most antidepressants cause weight gain by impacting how these neurochemicals affect eating behavior and energy expenditure (exercise and activity). Many of these antidepressants also raise cytokine levels, occasionally dramatically, and can even cause or precipitate diabetes.

These facts alone make a strong case for cytokine and brain happiness being connected. The future holds great promise for improved depression treatment and improved metabolism as we unravel these delicate chemical interactions.

What Results Could I Expect with MNT?

The symptoms of depression most likely to improve with MNT are fatigue (lack of energy), joy, motivation, and sex drive. Based on over a decade of clinical experience, these symptoms most dramatically improve during Food Phase 1 of the Plan.

The Plan is not a primary treatment of depression but it can aid or improve response to primary treatment.

Nurses, nutrition counselors, and other clinicians as well as your physician may play a supportive psychological role in depression treatment.

Because some antidepressant medications may contribute to weight gain and sexual dysfunction, it's important to talk to your doctor about how possible medication side effects might impact your general health. MNT may play a vital role in managing side effects that could occur with those medications that may best treat your depressive symptoms.

At the very least, the Amino Solution offers balanced nutrition for balanced brain function while reducing the levels of toxic cytokines known to be associated with depression. A lower, leaner weight will improve self confidence, make movement (exercise) easier, and will gain more favorable social interaction from others — factors all known to effect depression.

How Can I Measure Symptom Change with the Plan?

First, visit your physician to determine what might be causing your depression. Next, score the DOCTORdiet Psychological Profile (online at www.drdiet.com) prior to starting the Plan and rate your level of hopelessness in the Disease/Symptom Questionnaire on the next page. This will give you a baseline measurement of how depressed you feel.

Depression tends to come back (or relapse) if not completely resolved. The more frequent the relapse, the greater the chance you might suffer from chronic depression.

Most importantly, you (and your doctor) need a way to measure progress over time. Take the DOCTORdiet Psychological Profile again after Food Phase 1, and after twelve weeks (for those following the 7- or 14-day Plan). Re-score yourself every 12 weeks thereafter. Talk with your doctor at each regular visit about your symptoms and how they might change using the PrescriptFit™ Plan.

↞ Chapter 10: Enhancing Wellness with MNT ↠

As you progress through the Plan, note how you feel when adding each food category. If a particular food seems to be related to when you experience symptoms of depression, share this information with your doctor and use the knowledge you gain to modify your diet.

As with any medical condition, treatment may involve taking medications to reduce your depression symptoms. Many of these medications require close physician supervision to change the dose or stop taking them. With PrescriptFit™, you may find that as your symptoms lessen, you will need to take less medication OR perhaps discontinue your medications entirely.

Do not change how often or how much of your prescription medication you take without your doctor's approval; serious side effects or complications could result.

WHAT DO I NEED TO DO?

1. See your physician to determine what might be causing your symptoms. Talk with your doctor about incorporating MNT into your treatment plan.

2. Take the DOCTORdiet Psychological Profile before beginning the PrescriptFit Plan. Take the Profile again after Food Phase I and after 12 weeks on the Plan.

3. Record your symptoms of depression on the Disease/Symptom Questionnaire below on a scale of 0–10 with "0" being "none" and "10" being "thoughts of suicide." Be sure to record your discomfort level again at the end of each Food Phase or every four weeks.

4. Review the results with your doctor —talk about how you're feeling and changes in your need for prescription medications and doses prescribed based on MNT results.

DEPRESSION DISEASE/SYMPTOM QUESTIONNAIRE

DEPRESSION RATING*	None Thoughts of Suicide
	0 1 2 3 4 5 6 7 8 9 10

* COMPLETE THE DOCTORdiet PSYCHOLOGICAL PROFILE (ONLINE AT WWW.DRDIET.COM) AS DIRECTED; NEVER ALTER HOW YOU TAKE MEDICATIONS FOR DEPRESSION WITHOUT CONSULTING YOUR DOCTOR.

You should see your physician if you have any symptoms of breathlessness.

DYSPNEA (BREATHLESSNESS)

What is Dyspnea?

Dyspnea, or breathlessness, is any perceived difficulty breathing or pain you feel when breathing. It can be a symptom of many disorders, especially:

> Cardiac disease (coronary obstruction, CHF, valve disease, other)

> Pulmonary disease (asthma, emphysema, other)

> Kidney disease with edema (swelling)

> Liver disease with edema (swelling)

> Anemia (iron deficiency, B-12 deficiency, other)

> Hypothyroidism

What Causes Dyspnea?

Breathlessness may be caused by medical conditions or simply by excessive weight. Breathlessness may be a symptom of underlying cardiac disease. Physician evaluation is recommended, including a cardiac stress test and cardiac ultrasound exam. A chest x-ray is also indicated, especially in smokers.

If breathlessness resolves during Food Phase 1 or 2, cardiac causes are still possible. One would not expect breathlessness from excess weight to improve within 4 weeks of treatment, as only a minimal amount of weight would be lost relative to total needed to lose.

∾ Chapter 10: Enhancing Wellness with MNT ∾

What Role Might Cytokine Imbalance Play?

Cytokines are intimately involved with the function of small blood vessels and inflammation. Most of the conditions cited above have small blood vessel malfunction and/or inflammation as a primary component of the illness. While dyspnea is a symptom, it is related to cardiopulmonary function. Relaxing of the pulmonary (lung) small blood vessels and the small blood vessels downstream from the heart improve circulation, improve oxygen exchange, and therefore, improve dyspnea or breathlessness.

What Results Could I Expect with MNT?

Dyspnea improves very rapidly, in most cases, regardless of the primary cause (with the exception of emphysema). Most symptoms are measurably better in the first week. It's very reinforcing to track your ability to breathe better after each Plan phase. At the very least, improvement should be noted within four weeks. Breathlessness beyond this point is usually not improved by MNT.

Occasionally, a specific food may precipitate fluid retention, blood vessel spasm, or bronchial spasm leading to relapse of breathlessness. If breathlessness recurs when adding any specific food group, restart Food Phase 1 (with physician notification and supervision) and continue until symptoms resolve. Add the subsequent Food Phases slowly (every one to two weeks) and cautiously.

How Can I Measure Symptom Change on the Plan?

First, visit your physician to determine the cause of your breathlessness. Next, take a baseline measurement of the degree of discomfort you feel. Most importantly, you (and your doctor) need a way to measure progress over time. Talk with your doctor at each regular visit about your symptoms and how they might change using the Plan.

As with any medical condition, treatment may mean that you are taking medications to reduce your dyspnea symptoms. With this Plan, you may find that as your symptoms lessen, you will need to take less medication OR perhaps discontinue your medications entirely. If you are taking prescription medicines, talk to your doctor about when and how to cut down on what you take BEFORE you make any changes.

WHAT DO I NEED TO DO?

1. See your physician to determine what might be causing your symptoms. Talk with your doctor about incorporating MNT into your treatment plan, depending on what medical condition might be causing the symptoms.

2. Record your level of discomfort on the Disease/Symptom Questionnaire below on a scale of 0–10 with "0" being "never breathless" and "10" being "always breathless." Be sure to record your discomfort level again at the end of each Food Phase or every four weeks.

3. Review the results with your doctor — talk about how you're feeling and changes in your need for prescription medications and doses prescribed based on MNT results.

DYSPNEA (BREATHLESSNESS) DISEASE/SYMPTOM QUESTIONNAIRE

FREQUENCY OF BREATHLESSNESS	Never Always 0 1 2 3 4 5 6 7 8 9 10

* **WARNING:** DO NOT DISCONTINUE OR ALTER PRESCRIBED MEDICATIONS WITHOUT FIRST CONSULTING WITH YOUR DOCTOR.

∞ Chapter 10: Enhancing Wellness with MNT ∞

EDEMA (SWELLING)

What is Edema?

Edema is visible swelling in certain parts of the body, especially the feet and legs. This swelling occurs as a result of excess fluid accumulating under the skin in the spaces around blood vessels. Edema is a symptom of serious disease until proven otherwise, requiring complete medical evaluation and physician monitoring.

> Any undiagnosed edema requires physician evaluation.

What Causes Edema?

Edema can occur as a result of certain situations (e.g., being pregnant, prolonged standing, or long airplane rides), obesity, age, or injury. Certain conditions, such as "failure" of the heart, kidney, or liver, a blood clot in the leg, insulin resistance syndrome (IRS), varicose veins, burns, bites, malnutrition, or surgery, can cause swelling in one or both legs.

What Role Might Cytokines Play?

Fat tissue produces a cytokine protein (angiotensinogen) that causes salt retention. Synthesis or release of this protein can be induced by a single meal if high in calories, fat, and/or carbohydrates. Fluid retention is maintained chronically by continuing to eat a high-fat, high-sugar, high-calorie diet. Inflammatory cytokines damage small blood vessels and cause them to "leak" with resultant fluid retention. Cytokines also affect hormones secreted from the adrenal gland, heart, and brain that further promote fluid retention.

> Certain medications may also cause your legs to swell. These include hormones (especially estrogen and testosterone), blood-pressure-lowering drugs, arthritis medication (including cortisone), diabetic medication (especially glitazones — Actos® and Avandia®), steroids, and antidepressants (e.g.,, MAOIs).

What Results Could I Expect from MNT?

Edema from any cause typically responds to the MNT Plan, usually by Food Phases 1 or 2. Patients on diuretics (fluid pills) or vasodilators (heart or high blood pressure medication)

Close physician supervision is required for those taking fluid, high blood pressure, or heart medication (see hypertension and congestive heart failure discussions beginning on pages 176 and 203, respectively).

If you are taking prescription medicines, talk to you doctor about when and how to cut down on what you take BEFORE you make any changes.

should be very alert to hypotension (low blood pressure) in Food Phase 1 or 2. Rapid fluid loss may occur, requiring discontinuance of medication. After your edema subsides in Food Phase 1 and 2, stay alert for signs of relapse. Depending on cause, relapse may occur after a single meal of a higher fat, higher carbohydrate food or for other reasons (e.g., large salt intake, menstrual swelling, or certain arthritis medicine). Swelling should quickly resolve with resumption of Plan.

How Can I Measure Symptom Change on the Plan?

Talk with your doctor about what may be causing your swelling — cardiac illness, hypothyroidism, hypertension, OR perhaps a medication. If the latter, MNT will not reduce your symptoms; however, it can help determine if your edema is related to medication, depending on how quickly you see results without reducing medication dose or discontinuing altogether. Take a "baseline" measurement before beginning the Plan and again after each Food Phase or every four weeks.

WHAT DO I NEED TO DO?

1. Grade the level of swelling you have on a scale from 0–10 (with "0" being no swelling at all to a "10" being severe edema).
2. Be sure to check the symptoms and grade your swelling AGAIN at the end of each Food Phase or every four weeks.
3. Take the results with you to your next doctor's appointment. Talk about how you're feeling and whether or not medications or other factors may be related to your swelling.

EDEMA DISEASE/SYMPTOM QUESTIONNAIRE

LEVEL OF SWELLING	None Severe 0 1 2 3 4 5 6 7 8 9 10

* **WARNING:** KEEP IN CLOSE CONTACT WITH YOUR DOCTOR DURING INITIAL PHASES OF MNT; FLUID LOSS COULD REQUIRE IMMEDIATE MEDICATION CHANGE TO AVOID HYPOTENSION.

Chapter 10: Enhancing Wellness with MNT

Fatigue

What is Fatigue?

Fatigue, characterized as physical and/or mental weariness, occurs either as a symptom of illness or as a side effect of medication. Normal fatigue occurs as a result of exertion, stress, or dealing with illness (e.g., "fighting off a cold").

What Causes Fatigue?

Common, reversible causes of fatigue are sleep disorders, depression, cardiac disease, anemia, and hypothyroidism. High blood pressure, depression, antihistamines, sleeping, and anti-anxiety medications may also cause fatigue related side effects.

What Role Might Cytokine Imbalance Play?

Cytokines most likely impact fatigue via disturbances in brain function with resultant sleep disturbances, such as sleep apnea. Additional fatigue occurs when there is a malfunction in the cardiopulmonary system that results in restless sleep due to poor breathing. Finally, fatigue may be due to "stress" hormones (adrenalin and cortisone) induced by excess cytokine production in fat and liver cells. Improvement in symptoms is clearly related to improvement in "toxic" cytokine levels (TNF, IL-1 and IL-6, CRP, and others).

What Results Could I Expect with MNT?

Fatigue often responds to the MNT Plan, regardless of cause. It is also one of the symptoms to return quickly with overeating/weight gain.

As higher-calorie, higher-fat, and higher-carbohydrate Food Phases are added, a particular food group may be identified that produces increased fatigue, signally that a food group should be avoided.

If you are experiencing fatigue as a result of medications, MNT will not reduce your symptoms. However, MNT can help you and your doctor determine if your fatigue is related to medication. If you do not see results within the first few weeks, and are taking medication known for possible fatigue side effects, the chances are good that the medication is the culprit.

Fatigue is an important symptom to follow with each progressive Phase, typically responding to the first two Food Phases of the Plan.

How Can I Measure Symptom Change on the Plan?

First, you need to be clear about what may be causing your fatigue. Your physician may need to evaluate you for cardiac illness, hypothyroidism, anemia, or major depressive disorder.

Because many medications associated with fatigue side effects are prescribed for other conditions that respond to MNT, you and your doctor may find (over time) that your need for these medications will diminish. Take a baseline measurement of your fatigue and re-measure after each Food Phase or every four weeks.

Most importantly, you (and your doctor) need a way to measure progress over time. Talk with your doctor at each regular visit about your symptoms and how they might change using the Plan. If you are taking prescription medicines, talk to your doctor about when and how to cut down on what you take BEFORE you make any changes.

WHAT DO I NEED TO DO?

1. Grade the level of energy you have on a scale from 0–10 (with "0" being no energy at all to a "10" being high energy).
2. Be sure to check the symptoms and grade your fatigue AGAIN at the end of each Food Phase or every four weeks.
3. Take the results with you to your next doctor's appointment. Talk about how you're feeling and whether medications may be related to your fatigue.

FATIGUE DISEASE/SYMPTOM QUESTIONNAIRE

LEVEL OF FATIGUE	No energy High energy 0 1 2 3 4 5 6 7 8 9 10

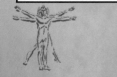

Chapter 10: Enhancing Wellness with MNT

Fibromyalgia

What is Fibromyalgia?

Fibromyalgia is a complex chronic condition of unknown origin that affects women far more than men (80-90 percent), and those typically over 20 years of age. The condition involves pain in the muscles and soft tissue for which no diagnostic test can determine cause (e.g., blood tests, x-rays, MRI, CAT scan, etc.) Muscle and bone surfaces are typically most tender. Although fibromyalgia does not appear to shorten one's lifespan nor necessarily be physically debilitating, it is highly recurrent — full recovery is rare. However, with good support and treatment (usually involving some medication, good sleep habits, and exercise), fibromyalgia will not severely damage quality of life.

Those with fibromyalgia tend to suffer from sleep disorders, depression, and anxiety.

What Causes Fibromyalgia?

We really know very little about fibromyalgia; however, many theories exist regarding its cause. Some believe that the disorder is linked to viral infection, psychological disturbances or trauma, altered pain perception, lack of growth hormone, or lack of exercise. Other researchers point to change in sleep patterns or low levels of serotonin — a hormone that regulates moods and sleep. Research has shown that people with fibromyalgia tend to have disturbances in their deep sleep and different serotonin levels than others.

Female hormones are known to affect many brain and nerve neurotransmitters, including pain-mediating ones.

Because of the prevalence among women (90% of those diagnosed), experts believe that the disorder is related in some way to female hormones.

The Amino Solution
©2009 Stanford A. Owen, MD

What Role Might Cytokine Imbalance Play?

Scientists point to Substance P (also known as neurokephlin) as a chemical in our bodies that modifies pain sensation in nerve fibers and brain cells. Research indicates that Substance P abnormalities may effect depression and are abnormal in fibromyalgia. Because cytokines produced by fat cells influence production and function of Substance P, and female hormones regulate fat cell physiology, this link between obesity, cytokines, hormones, and pain regulation is very plausible.

What Results Could I Expect with MNT?

Cases of fibromyalgia improve, and even resolve, using the PrescriptFit™ MNT Plan, although response is difficult to predict. Most cases improve by Phase 1 or 2, especially when using the 7- or 14-day Food Phase Plan. You should see a change in symptoms by the end of week 4 if you rigidly adhere to the Plan.

Most patients experience improved sleep (and less fatigue) the quickest, followed by improved mood. Pain usually improves after sleep improves.

How Can I Measure Symptom Change on the Plan?

Learn what may be causing your muscle pain and other symptoms. Visit your physician to determine whether you have fibromyalgia. Talk with your doctor about MNT and its impact on sleep, fatigue, depression, and other symptoms you're experiencing. Next, you want to have measurement of how severe each symptom is for you. This will give you a "baseline" to compare with future measurements.

⌁ Chapter 10: Enhancing Wellness with MNT ⌁

Most importantly, you (and your doctor) need a way to measure progress over time. Talk with your doctor at each regular visit about your symptoms and how they might change using the Plan.

As with any medical condition, treatment traditionally means taking medications to reduce symptoms. You may find that as your symptoms lessen with MNT, you will need to take less medication OR perhaps discontinue pain medications entirely. If you are taking prescription medicines, talk to you doctor about when and how to cut down on what you take BEFORE you make any changes.

WHAT DO I NEED TO DO?

1. Check each symptom you are currently experiencing in the Disease/ Symptom Questionnaire below.
2. Grade the level of pain you have on a scale from 0–10 (with "0" being no symptom at all to a "10" being severe and constant discomfort), as well as, how often you need medication for the pain.
3. Next, rate how you sleep (with "0" being "never sleep well" to "10," which indicates that you "always sleep well."
4. Be sure to check the symptoms and grade your level of discomfort/sleep satisfaction AGAIN at the end of each Food Phase or every four weeks.
5. Take the results with you to your next doctor's appointment. Talk about how you're feeling and whether you still need any prescription medications for fibromyalgia.
6. Note if symptoms relapse with subsequent Food Phases or with off-Plan eating.

FIBROMYALGIA DISEASE/SYMPTOM QUESTIONNAIRE

Symptom Experience	Level of Discomfort
PAIN	None Severe/Constant 0 1 2 3 4 5 6 7 8 9 10
SLEEP	Never Well Always Well 0 1 2 3 4 5 6 7 8 9 10

* WARNING: NEVER DISCONTINUE A PHYSICIAN-PRESCRIBED MEDICATION WITHOUT CONSULTING WITH YOUR DOCTOR

The Amino Solution
©2009 Stanford A. Owen, MD

INFERTILITY

What is Infertility?

Infertility is a complex disorder that occurs in both men and women. It is a disease of the reproductive system that prevents conception and can occur because of problems with any facet of the reproductive process.

What Causes Infertility?

For women, most infertility cases stem from some problem with ovulation. Each step of the process from egg maturation to implantation may be influenced by dietary factors. There is an apparent relationship between infertility and obesity, especially in those who have insulin resistance syndrome (IRS).

What Role Might Cytokine Imbalance Play?

In the early 1990s, researchers discovered a hormone produced by fat cells — leptin — that helps regulate food intake and metabolism as well as fat storage in the cells. Subsequently, leptin was found to play a role in fertility. As excess nutrition and obesity develop, especially in insulin-resistant individuals, "resistance" to the action of leptin also develops.

What Results Could I Expect from MNT?

Although the link between MNT and fertility is not clear-cut, there appears to be one: Women with IRS (insulin resistant syndrome) are especially likely to benefit from MNT, partially because polycystic ovary syndrome is characterized, possibly even caused, by insulin resistance. Additionally, obesity influences leptin, a hormone important in regulating the entire process of conception.

See page 180 through 184 for discussion and disease/symptom tracking information for IRS.

Although the link between cytokines and Leptin has not been definitely established, the combination of weight loss and cytokine balance appears to be critical to positively influencing conception.

In addition to other possible hormonal and cytokine influences, Leptin influences brain hormones involved in development, fertilization, and implantation of the egg as well as growth of the placenta.

Chapter 10: Enhancing Wellness with MNT

Virtually every obese woman treated in our clinic for infertility with MNT has conceived within three months, indicating that "the diet" and not "the obesity" contributed to the infertility. Women who are amennorrheic (without periods) typically resume menstrual periods within the first eight weeks with rigid adherence to Food Phases 1 and 2 of the Plan.

With MNT, those who are overweight as well as those who have IRS, polycystic ovary syndrome, or diabetes are the most likely to see results.

How Can I Measure Symptom Change on the Plan?

First of all, infertile couples should undergo evaluation by a fertility specialist prior to considering the PrescriptFit™ MNT Plan to determine possible causes and treatment solutions. Talk to the specialist about trying MNT prior to medication or other therapies.

Unlike other illnesses discussed in this section, there is no Disease/ Symptom Questionnaire for infertility. The important measurement is to pinpoint ovulation in one of the ways discussed at left.

Fertilization can best occur two weeks following a menstrual period when the woman ovulates. To better pinpoint when ovulation occurs, women can use:

1. **Calendar tracking** — Record past menstrual cycle start date and duration to determine when you are most likely to be fertile.

If appropriate, use the 14-day/phase Plan for best chances of fertility.

2. **Taking basal body temperature** — Use a basal thermometer to check your body temperature each morning before becoming active. A rise of 0.4 to 1 degree Fahrenheit occurs when you ovulate.

3. **Checking vaginal mucus** — Daily test vaginal mucus for color (yellow, white, clear or cloudy), consistency (thick, sticky, or stretchy), and feel (dry, wet, sticky, slippery, stretchy). Ovulation probably occurs the same day that your mucus is clearest, most slippery, and most stretchy.

Regular ovulation will not ensure conception. It is, however, a vital starting point. Work with your fertility specialist to optimize all the factors necessary to become pregnant.

INSOMNIA

What is Insomnia?

Insomnia and sleep apnea (see pages 188–190) are different conditions. Insomnia typically means that the person has difficulty falling asleep or staying asleep, with or without subsequent daytime sleepiness. Those with sleep apnea typically experience daytime sleepiness despite being "asleep" all night.

People who suffer from insomnia get either too little sleep or the sleep they get is not very restful and refreshing. The problem doesn't necessarily have anything to do with the number of hours you sleep at night; it has to do with the quality of that sleep. For some, the problem is having trouble falling asleep in the first place. For others, the chronic tiredness comes from waking up too early in the morning. Some people fall asleep with no trouble, but wake up several times during the night and struggle to get back to sleep.

No matter what the pattern, insomnia leaves you feeling tired, sometimes even after "sleeping" seven to eight hours. This lack of adequate rest causes problems during the day: excessive sleepiness, fatigue, trouble thinking clearly or staying focused, or feeling depressed/irritable.

What Causes Insomnia?

Underlying medical causes of insomnia include:

- Chronic medical conditions, such as cancer, asthma, or arthritis
- Mental disorders, such as depression, anxiety, or bipolar disorder
- Hyperthyroidism (an overactive thyroid)
- Diabetes
- Anemia (from deficiencies in iron or B-12)
- Trouble breathing because of EITHER sleep apnea OR acid reflux with aspiration of food contents into the lungs
- Alzheimer's disease

Insomnia may be a temporary problem induced by situational stress at home or at work, having a poor sleep environment (too much light, noise, or a partner who snores), or even certain medications. This type of short-term or occasional insomnia can last from a single night to a few weeks or occur from time to time.

If insomnia persists for at least three nights a week for over a month or more, you should see your physician about possible underlying medical causes. If this is not the case, your physician can help you identify patterns (working erratic shifts, not exercising, drinking caffeine or alcohol too close to bedtime, etc.) that might help positively alter your sleep patterns.

What Role Might Cytokine Imbalance Play?

How MNT improves insomnia is unknown. A majority of patients presenting to our clinic complain of insomnia. A majority improve sleep when following the Plan. Some improvement may be due to other related medical conditions, such as sleep apnea, acid reflux, or even improved oxygen exchange from better blood flow. No specific cytokines have been related to general insomnia related to anxiety. Perhaps, improved metabolism related to balanced cytokine production (see other disease sections) lowers adrenalin and cortisone levels, which are known to aggravate insomnia.

What Results Could I Expect with MNT?

Those suffering from insomnia often note improvement on the MNT Plan. Why this occurs is unknown; however, we suspect that improved brain function is related to improved nutrition or improved metabolism. Also, we know that branched-chain amino acids benefit patients suffering from a number of conditions that cause insomnia (depression, acid reflux, sleep apnea, arthritis, etc.), and not getting enough restful sleep complicates these conditions. Because of this interplay, you don't know if your insomnia got better because your arthritis symptoms eased (for example), or whether your arthritis symptoms improved because you're finally getting a good night's rest on a regular basis.

How Can I Measure Symptom Change on the Plan?

As with any medical condition, treatment may involve taking medications to reduce symptoms. You may find that as your symptoms lessen, you will need to take less medication OR perhaps discontinue your medications entirely. If you are taking prescription medicines, talk to you doctor about when and how to cut down on what you take BEFORE you make any changes.

First, you need to be clear about what might be causing your insomnia. Talk to your doctor about your medical and sleep history. Find out if there's an underlying medical problem that needs attention.

If you have chronic insomnia, you will want to measure how severe each symptom is for you. This will give you a "baseline" to compare with future measurements. Most importantly, you (and your doctor) need a way to measure progress over time. Measure your symptoms again after four weeks or following each food phase. Take the results to your doctor and discuss how your symptoms have changed using the Plan.

WHAT DO I NEED TO DO?

1. Rate each symptom you are currently experiencing in the Disease/ Symptom Questionnaire below, noting how long it takes to fall asleep initially as well as how long you sleep before waking and then struggle to get back to sleep.
2. Be sure to check the symptoms and rate your level of sleeplessness AGAIN at the end of each Food Phase or every four weeks.
3. Take the results with you to your next doctor's appointment. Talk about how you're feeling and whether or not you still need any medications or other lifestyle changes to reduce your insomnia.

INSOMNIA DISEASE/SYMPTOM QUESTIONNAIRE

Symptom Experience	Level of Discomfort							
DIFFICULTY FALLING ASLEEP	AVERAGE MINUTES TO FALL ASLEEP							
	1	5	10	15	30	60	120	180
TIMES AWAKENED AFTER INITIAL SLEEP ESTABLISHED	NUMBER OF INSTANCES							
	1	2	3	4	5	6	7	8
LENGTH OF TIME TO REESTABLISH SLEEP	AVERAGE MINUTES							
	1	5	10	15	30	60	120	180

The Amino Solution
©2009 Stanford A. Owen, MD

Chapter 10: Enhancing Wellness with MNT

JOINT PAIN (HIP, KNEE, FEET)

What is Joint Pain?

Joint pain in the hip, knee, or feet all typically occur in those who are obese. The joints associated with these areas bear the weight of our frame and help to keep us upright. Stress on these joints, as our bodies adapt to changes in weight and body shape, can often lead to debilitating discomfort.

The most common joint complaint is **knee pain.** The knee bears the brunt of increased weight and abnormal angle-stress from obesity. The knee is also subject to sudden twists and bends of unexpected slips and falls. This is often a problem for those who are obese and perhaps not as agile or flexible due to the excess weight. Minor tears in the ligaments, tendons, and cartilage (that result from these slips and falls) promote inflammation and swelling.

Foot pain is a frequent complaint of obese patients. Foot pain can arise from the ankle joint, the nerves to the foot, and ligaments (plantar fasciitis or heel spur). All three conditions are more common in obesity for the same reasons noted with knee pain. The human foot was designed to bear weight down the shank of the leg and heel, rather than towards the toes (as it must do in obesity because of having a larger abdomen).

Hip pain is the least frequent and most severe type of joint damage related to obesity. Pain from the hip joint is typically felt on the front of the hip. Hip pain requires expert diagnosis and rehab; you will need to see a joint specialist and possibly a physical therapist as well.

Be sure to see a physician familiar with foot pain for accurate diagnosis.

The Amino Solution
©2009 Stanford A. Owen, MD

What Causes Joint Pain?

Joint pain and obesity are bedfellows. Joint pain may occur from increased strain and tearing of joint support (ligament, tendon, cartilage, bone) due to excessive weight and from abnormal joint angles from distorted weight distribution.

On another level, joint pain is related to your body's ability to repair damaged collagen — the support protein for the ligaments, tendons, cartilage, and bone. Obesity is associated with changes in your body's hormone levels — the ones that impact your ability to repair collagen. Those who are obese tend to have low testosterone levels and low growth hormone levels, both of which are essential to collagen repair. Obesity is also associated with elevated levels of cortisone, which destroys collagen. As we age, our ability to repair damaged collagen also decreases, making obesity and aging a very troubling combination.

What Role Might Cytokine Imbalance Play?

Fat cells produce cytokines that promote immune inflammation that damages joint structures. The combination of increased weight, abnormal angles of movement, and increased immune damage with diminished collagen repair destroys joints and causes pain with disability. Those who are obese have more problems with joint injury because their bodies produce too much of a protein enzyme (metalloproteases) that destroys collagen. Since overproduction of this enzyme is linked to out-of-balance cytokines, PrescriptFit™ can offer significant benefits.

~ Chapter 10: Enhancing Wellness with MNT ~

What Results Could I Expect with MNT?

Knee pain often improves with the MNT Plan via decreased weight and diminished inflammation. In our clinic, decreased pain and medication requirements are seen long before major weight changes. Expert rehabilitation is vital. Abdominal weakness is just as important as obesity in promoting abnormal knee-angle stress. "Ab" strengthening should be a practiced daily in those with back, hip, knee, or foot pain.

For improving **foot pain**, the Plan fosters weight loss and positive changes to posture that occur with reducing abdomen size. In addition, exercise and physical therapy as well as heel pads and arch supports will likely speed recovery. In our clinic, those using the MNT Plan often note improvement in foot pain, although usually at a slower rate than those experiencing improvement in knee pain.

How Can I Measure Symptom Change on the Plan?

First, you need to be clear about what might be causing your joint pain. Talk to your doctor about the type of pain you have, when you first noticed it, the severity, and what treatment combination might be best for you. Next, you want to have a measurement of how severe the joint pain is for you. This will give you a "baseline" to compare with future measurements.

Most importantly, you (and your doctor) need a way to measure progress over time. Talk with your doctor at each regular visit about your symptoms and how they might change using the Plan.

Those with **hip pain** are probably less likely to improve using the Plan. However, diminished weight and decreased abdominal protuberance helps all joints below the pelvis.

As with any medical condition, treatment traditionally means taking medications to reduce symptoms. A number of prescription and over-the-counter pain medications can be taken to reduce symptoms. You may find that as your symptoms lessen, you will need to take less medication OR perhaps discontinue your medications entirely. If you are taking prescription medicines, talk to your doctor about when and how to cut down on what you take BEFORE you make any changes.

WHAT DO I NEED TO DO?

1. Using the Disease/Symptom Questionnaire below, indicate for each type of joint pain you have (knee, foot, hip) the severity initially on a scale from 0–10 (with "0" being no symptom at all to a "10" being severe discomfort).

2. Be sure to check the symptoms and grade your level of discomfort AGAIN at the end of each 12 weeks.

3. Record the number of medications you currently take for each type of joint pain initially when beginning MNT and again after 12 weeks.

4. Take the results with you to your next doctor's appointment. Talk about how you're feeling and whether or not you still need to take medications for joint pain.

JOINT PAIN DISEASE/SYMPTOM QUESTIONNAIRE

INITIAL KNEE PAIN	KNEE PAIN AT 12 WEEKS
MILD SEVERE 1 2 3 4 5 6 7 8 9 10	MILD SEVERE 1 2 3 4 5 6 7 8 9 10
INITIAL FOOT PAIN	FOOT PAIN AT 12 WEEKS
MILD SEVERE 1 2 3 4 5 6 7 8 9 10	MILD SEVERE 1 2 3 4 5 6 7 8 9 10
INITIAL HIP PAIN	HIP PAIN AT 12 WEEKS
MILD SEVERE 1 2 3 4 5 6 7 8 9 10	MILD SEVERE 1 2 3 4 5 6 7 8 9 10

Number of Medications Used _____ (e.g., Tylenol™ + Ibuprofen = 2)

* **WARNING:** NEVER DISCONTINUE A PHYSICIAN-PRESCRIBED MEDICATION WITHOUT CONSULTING WITH YOUR DOCTOR.

The Amino Solution
©2009 Stanford A. Owen, MD

NOTES

NOTES

_____
_____
_____
_____
_____
_____
_____
_____
_____
_____
_____
_____
_____
_____
_____
_____
_____
_____
_____
_____
_____
_____
_____
_____
_____
_____
_____
_____
_____
_____
_____
_____
_____
_____
_____

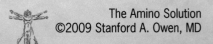

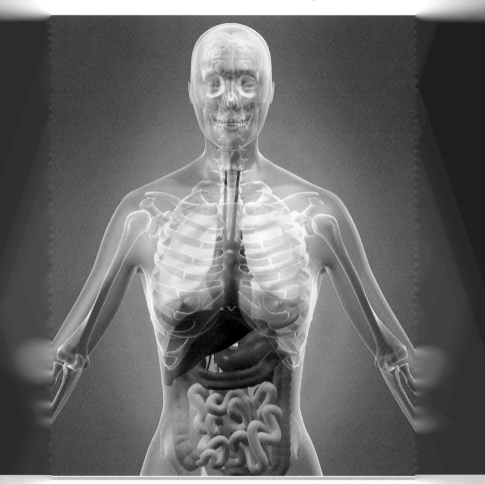

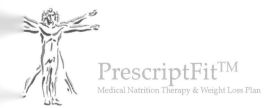

PrescriptFit™
Medical Natrition Therapy & Weight Loss Plan

The key to why the Amino Solution works to reduce disease symptoms and promote weight loss lies in the relationship between fat cells, cytokines, and branched chain amino acids. Below are some definitions to help you understand these relationships. Be sure to talk to your doctor about cytokines and the impact of fat cells on your overall health.

ADIPOKIN

See pages 234 through 235 for a list of common adipokins and their functions.

A cytokine produced by adipose (fat) cells. A short list of known adipokins includes adiponectin, resistin, leptin, tumor necrosis factor, angiotensinogen, interleukin 1,2,6,18, plasminogen activator inhibitor–1 (PAI–1), macrophage inhibiting factor, adipsin, free fatty acids, and growth factors.

BRANCHED CHAIN AMINO ACIDS

Leucine, Isoleucine, and Valine are the primary branched chain amino acids. They are called "branched" due to their chemical structure. These amino acids, plus threonine and lysine, comprise 75% of amino acids used for energy metabolism or protein synthesis. The ratio of each amino acid affects the metabolism of other amino acids. Therefore, achieving balance of the key amino acids can improve energy and protein metabolism.

CYTOKINES

Protein molecules (peptides) made by cells of the immune system, fat cells, and other organs that regulate inflammation, metabolism, cell growth, vascular tone, blood cell formation, and behavior. Cytokines made by fat cells are called "adipokines" (from an adipose cell). Key characteristics of cytokines are that they:

- **Have multiple functions:** The same cytokine may regulate inflammation, blood vessel function, or infertility.

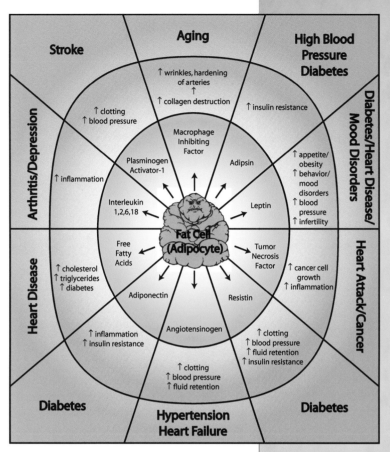

- **Are redundant:** Different cytokines may have the same function.

- **Work in a cascading manner:** One cytokine released may trigger the next, then another, and another, resulting in many different reactions in different organs.

- **May come from different organs:** Multiple organs make the same cytokines (e.g., leptin may be made by fat cells, brain tissue, or the intestine).

The Amino Solution
©2009 Stanford A. Owen, MD

Common Adipokins

Adiponectin
A prevalent and protective cytokine — Higher levels of adiponectin prevent heart disease and diabetes. Lower levels are produced by obesity, high fat, high sugar diets, inactivity, and inflammation from other diseases (arthritis).

Adipsin
Made by abdominal fat cells, this cytokine promotes insulin resistance and fluid retention. It also activates other inflammatory cytokines.

Angiotensinogen
A cytokine that regulates blood pressure and fluid balance, inflammation of blood vessels, and growth of fat cells.

Growth Factors
A host of cytokines that make cells grow (including cancer cells). Epidermal growth factor produces thickening of skin cells, especially on the neck and arm pits, causing darkening of the skin (acanthosis nigricans) and skin tags.

Free Fatty Acids (FFA)
Triglycerides released by fat cells that float to the liver or muscle and are used as energy. When excess FFA is formed, it causes insulin resistance, muscle malfunction, and cytokine formation.

Interleukin 1, 2, 6, and 18
Cytokines that regulate inflammation and immune function. Levels rise with obesity, high fat, high sugar diets, and other diseases of inflammation.

Leptin

The first discovered adipokine — Leptin regulates eating behavior, blood vessel function, immune function, fertility, and at least 30 other functions.

Macrophage Inhibiting Factor (MIF)

A cytokine that promotes macrophage (white blood cells that ingest foreign material) attack on arteries and into fat tissue.

Plasminogen Activator Inhibitor-1 (PAI-1)

Cytokine that promotes clotting and thrombosis. Increases in obesity, high fat, high sugar diets. PAI-1 levels can reduce by 50% in one week on VLCD (very low calorie diets).

Resistin

Cytokine with opposite effects of adiponectin — Resistin causes "resistance" to the action of insulin in cell function.

Tumor Necrosis Factor (TNF)

A cytokine that regulates inflammation and immune function, including cancer control. TNF has a role in energy balance, insulin resistance and diabetes, fat metabolism, and blood vessel damage. Obesity and high-fat, high-sugar diets increase levels and function of TNF. Elevated TNF lowers adiponectin levels.

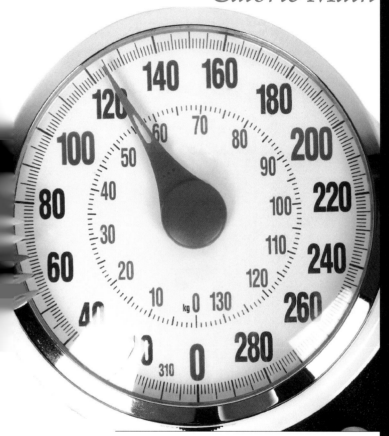

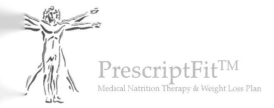

PrescriptFit™
Medical Nutrition Therapy & Weight Loss Plan

Calorie Math

Use the notes page at the end of this appendix to list those foods that you like (or are willing to experiment with) that "add up" to be the best "bang for your calorie buck."

Review the chart below and on the following page to see how the foods you eat "add up" to extra exercise in order to burn those calories. For example, is having fried shrimp rather than shrimp cocktail worth an extra mile of walking for every ounce you eat? Do the math; it will be a real eye-opener!

Food Item	Calories/ Ounce	# Ounces = 1 Mile of Walking
Beef	100–125	.75–1
Pork	100–150	.5–1
Seafood (grilled, baked, etc.)	25–30	4
Seafood (fried)	125	.75
Poultry (skinless, not fried)	50	2
Poultry (skin on)	75–100	1–1.25
Poultry (fried)	100–125	.75–1
Eggs (EACH)	1 Egg = 100	1 Egg = 1 Mile
Nuts	175	.57
Fruits lemon, tomato melon apple, pineapple, orange grapes banana avocado dried fruit	 5 10 15 20 30 45 85	 20 10 9 5 3 2 1–1.2
Snacks/Baked Goods chips bread muffins/cereal pastries/cake pie	 125–150 80 100 125 150	 .5–.75 1–1.2 1 .75 .5

Food Item	Calories/Cup	# Cups = 1 Mile of Walking
Beverages		
soft drinks (sweetened)	12	8–9
beer	12	8–9
wine	20	5
liquor (scotch, rum, etc.)	60	1.67
liqueur (brandy, kahlua, etc.)	100–150	.5–1
juice/whole milk	20	5
Dairy		
non-fat cottage cheese	25	4
yogurt	25–50	2–4
sour cream	30–50	2–4
cream cheese	50–75	2–2.5
cheese	25–100	1–4
ice cream	125–150	.5–.75
milk	20	5
cream	75	1.25
Vegetables		
leafy, green (bell pepper, celery, lettuce, summer squash)	10–20	5–10
onions, carrots, asparagus, okra, green beans, cauliflower, broccoli	40–60	2–3
winter squash, peas (fresh), stewed tomatoes, beans, diced potatoes	80–120	.8–1.25
corn, mashed potatoes, rice, dried peas, beans	140–200	.5–.71

* *One mile of walking/day (15 minutes) burns approximately 100 calories in a 150-pound individual.*

The Amino Solution
©2009 Stanford A. Owen, MD

NOTES

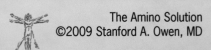

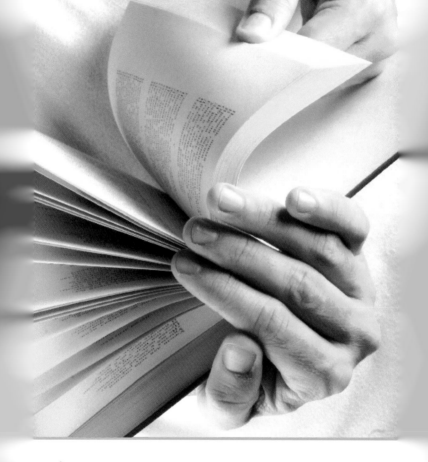

Appendix C
Suggested Reading for You and Your Doctor

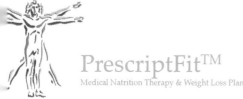

PrescriptFit™
Medical Nutrition Therapy & Weight Loss Plan

Resources for You

The Wellness Encyclopedia of Food and Nutrition by Sheldon Margen, M.D. and UC Berkeley; 512 pages; Random House, Inc.

The Mount Sinai School of Medicine Complete Book of Nutrition edited by Victor Herbert, M.D. and Genell J. Subak-Sharpe, M.S.; 796 pages; St. Martin's Press.

Complete Food and Nutrition Guide, 2nd ed. by Roberta Larson Duyff, MS, RD, FADA, CFCS; 672 pages; the American Dietetic Association (http://www.eatright.org/cps/rde/xchg/ada/hs.xsl/nutrition.html).

Cooking Light (http://www.cookinglight.com/cooking/cookbook) — Be sure to check out the annuals, *The Best of Cooking Light, The Cook's Essential Recipe Collection, CL Light and Easy; CL Holiday;* and *CL 5 Ingredients 15 Minute Cookbook* as well as those by Susan McIntosh (*CL Desserts Cookbook; CL Lose Weight Cookbook; CL Regional Fare Cookbook; CL Vegetarian Cookbook; CL Chicken Cookbook; CL Pasta Cookbook*). All are published by Oxmoor House.

The American Heart Association cookbooks (http://www. deliciousdecisions.org/) — Look for the *AHA Low Calorie Cookbook* and *Low-Fat, Low-Cholesterol Cookbook.*

Joslin Diabetes Healthy Carbohydrates Cookbook by Bonnie Sanders Polin, PhD and the staff of Joslin Diabetes Center; 288 pages; Fireside Publisher.

To better understand cytokines and their impacts on your health, look at these articles from *Time* and *Newsweek* Web site archives:

- "When the Body Attacks Itself" by Anne Underwood, *Newsweek*, December 8th, 15th, 2003, available at no cost to *Newsweek* subscribers only.

- "The Fires Within" by Christine Gorman, *Time Magazine*, February, 2004; available free at http://www.time.com/time/magazine/article/0,9171,993419,00.html.

Easy Healthy Dinners by Dan Rosenberg/Grand Avenue Books; 256 pages; Meredith Books.

Eating for Life by Bill Phillips; 405 pages; High Point Media, LLC.

EatingWell: Healthy in a Hurry Cookbook: 150 Delicious Recipes for Simple, Everyday Suppers in 45 Minutes or Less by Jim Romanoff and the editors of *EatingWell*; 256 pages; Countryman Press.

The Essential EatingWell Cookbook: Good Carbs, Good Fats, Great Flavors edited by Patsy Jamieson; *EatingWell*; 146 pages; Countryman Press.

Free recipes are also available online from a variety of product manufacturers, including:

- http://www.mollymcbutter.com/
- http://www.butterbuds.com/recipes/search.php
- http://splenda.allrecipes.com/Default.aspx
- http://www.mrsdash.com/MDrecipes/recipes_landing.cfm
- http://www.benecol.com/recipes/index.jhtml?id=benecol/recipes/re_main.inc
- http://www.chefpaul.com/recipes.html

RESOURCES FOR YOUR DOCTOR

The Role of Nutritional Supplements with Essential Amino Acids in Patients with Cardiovascular Disease and Diabetes Mellitus, Gheorghiade M, Dioguardi FS, Scognamiglio R, eds. *Am J Cardiol.* 2004;93(suppl):1A–46A.

Taylor V, MacQueen G. Associations between bipolar disorder and metabolic syndrome: a review. *J Clin Psychiatry.* 2006;67:1034–41.

Hinault C, Van Obberghen E, Mothe-Satney I. Role of amino acides in insulin signaling in adipocytes and their potential to decrease insulin resistance of adipose tissue. *J Nutr Biochem.* 2006 (Jun);17(6):374–8. Epub 2006 Apr 27.

Kane, P. Understanding the biochemical and biobehavioral nexus of depression. *Explore.* 1997;8(1). Accessed in December, 2006 at http://www.explorepub.com/articles/nutrition2.html.

Parker G, Gibson NA, Brotchie H, et al. Omega-3 fatty acids and mood disorders. *Am J Psychiatry.* 2006:163 (June):969–78.

Agras WS. Treatment of binge-eating disorder. In: Gabbard GO, ed. *Treatments of Psychiatric Disorders.* Washington, DC: American Psychiatric Press; 2001: 2209–19.

Alaswad K, LavieCJ, Milani RV, O'Keefe JH Jr. Fish oil in cardiovascular prevention. *The Ochsner Journal* 2002;4:83–91.

Alberti KG, Zimmet PZ. Definition, diagnosis and classification of diabetes mellitus and its complications: Part 1: diagnosis and classification of diabetes mellitus provisional report of a WHO consultation. *Diabet Med.* 1998;15:539–53.

American Association of Clinical Endocrinologists. The American Association of Clinical Endocrinologists medical guidelines for the management of diabetes mellitus: the AACE system of intensive diabetes self-management — 2002 update. *Endocr Pract.* 2002;8:40–82.

American Psychiatric Association. *Diagnostic and Statistical Manual of Mental Disorders. 4th ed.* Washington, DC: American Psychiatric Association; 1994:25–35, 78–85.

Anderson RE, Crespo CJ. Relationship between body weight gain and significant knee, hip, and back pain in older Americans. *Obes Res.* 2003;11(10):1159–62.

Ballenger JC, Davidson JR, Lecrubier Y, et al. Consensus statement on depression, anxiety, and cardiovascular disease. *J Clin Psychiatr.* 2001;62(suppl 8):24–7.

Baptista T, Veauliue S. Are leptin and cytokines involved in body weight gain during treatment with antipsychotic drigs? *Can J Psychiatry.* 2002;47:742–9.

Bard RL, Kalsi H. Effect of carotid atherosclerosis screening on risk stratification during primary cardiovascular disease prevention; *Am J Cardiol.* 2004 (April 15);93:1030–3.

Barefoot JC, Heitmann BL, Helms MJ, et al. Symptoms of depression and changes in body weight from adolescence to mid-life. *Int J Obes Relat Metab Disord.* 1998;22:688–94.

Bartlik B, Goldberg J. Female sexual arousal disorder. In: *Principles and Practice of Sex Therapy (3rd ed.),* S. R. Leiblum & R. C. Rosen (Eds.). 2000. New York: Guilford: pp. 85–117.

Becker JB, Breedlove MS, Crews D. *Behavioral Endocrinology.* 1992. Providence, RI: Bradford Press.

Beltowski J, Wojcicka G, Jamroz A. Stimulatory effect of leptin on nitric oxide production is impaired in dietary-induced obesity. *Obes Res.* 2003 (Dec); 11(12):1571–80.

Berne C, Pollare T, Lithell H. Effects of antihypertensive treatment on insulin sensitivity with special reference to ACE inhibitors. *Diabetes Care.* 1991;14:39–47.

Bickel C. Relation of markers of inflammation (CRP, fibrinogen, von Willebrand factor, and leukocyte count) and statin therapy to long-term mortality in patients with angiographically proven coronary artery disease. *Am J Cardiol.* 2002;89(4):901–4.

Bo S, Ganbino R, Dagani A, et al. Relationships between human serum resistin, inflammatory markers and insulin resistance. *Int. J Obes (Lond).* 2005 (Nov);29(11):1315–20.

Brook RD, Bard RL. Effect of short-term weight loss on the metabolic syndrome and conduit vascular endothelial function in overweight adults; *Am J Cardiol.* 2004(Apr. 15);93:1012–16.

Brunner EJ, Hemingway H, Walker BR, et al. Adrenocortical, autonomic, and inflammatory causes of the metabolic syndrome: nested case control study. *Circulation.* 2002;106:2659–65.

Caan B, Quesenberry C, Stolshek B, et al. Increases in pharmacy costs among obese members in an HMO. *Obes Res.* 1999;7:54s (abstract 0146).

Cabollero E. Endothelial dysfunction in obesity and insulin resistance: a road to diabetes and heart disease. *Obes Res. 2003* (Nov);11(11):1278–89.

Carpenter KM, Hasin DS, Allison DB, Faith MS. Relationships between obesity and DSM-IV major depressive disorder, suicide ideation, and suicide attempts: results from a general population study. *Am J Public Health.* 2000;90:251–7.

Ceddia RB. Direct metabolic regulation in skeletal muscle and fat tissue by leptin: implications for glucose and fatty acid homeostasis. *Int J Obes.* 2005 (Oct);29(10):1175–83.

Clark MG, Wallis MG, Barrett EJ,et al. Blood flow and muscle metabolism: a focus on insulin action. *Am J Physiol Endolcrinol Metab.* 2003 (Feb);284(2):E241–58.

Clifton PM, Keogh JB. Effect of weight loss on inflammatory and endothelial markers. *Int J Obesity.* 2005 (Dec);29(12):1445–51.

Crow S, Kendall D, Praus B, Thuras P. Binge eating and other psychopathology in patients with type II diabetes mellitus. *Int J Eat Disord.* 2001;30:222–26.

de Zwaan M, Mitchell JE, Raymond NC, et al. Binge-eating disorder: clinical features and treatment of a new diagnosis. *Harv Rev Psychiatry.* 1994;1:310–25.

DeBusk RF. Sexual activity in patients with angina. *JAMA.* 2003 (Dec);290(23):3129–33.

Diabetes Prevention Program Research Group. Reduction in the incidence of type 2 diabetes with lifestyle intervention or metformin. *N Engl J Med.* 2002;346:393–403.

Dioguardi, FS. Wasting and the substrate-to-energy controlled pathway: a role for insulin resistance and amino acids. *Am J Cardiol, Excerpta Medica*: April 2004.

Dixon JB, Dixon ME, O'Brien PE. Depression in association with severe obesity. *Archives of Internal Medicine.* 2003 (Sept. 22);163:2058–62.

Duffy SJ, Keaney JF Jr., Holbrook M, et al. Short- and long-term black tea consumption reverses endothelial dysfunction in patients with coronary artery disease. *Circulation.* 2001 (July 10);104:151–6.

Duncan BB, Schmidt MI, Chambless LE, et al. Inflammation markers predict increased weight gain in smoking quitters. *Obes Res.* 2003;11(11):1339–44.

Expert Panel on Detection, Evaluation, and Treatment of High Blood Cholesterol in Adults. Executive Summary of The Third Report of The National Cholesterol Education Program (NCEP). *JAMA.* 2001;285:2486–97.

Fain JN, Madan AK. Regulation of monocyte chemoattractant protein 1 (MCP-1) release by explants of human visceral adipose tissue. *Int. J Obes.* 2005 (Nov.);29(11):1299–1307.

Ford ES, Mokdad AH. Trends in waist circumference among U.S. adults. *Obes Res.* 2003;11(10):1123–1231.

Foster, GD, Wadden TA. Primary care physician's attitudes about obesity and its treatment. *Obes Res.* 2003;11(10):1168–77.

Garnett WR. Clinical pharmacology of topiramate: a review. *Epilepsia.* 2000;41(Suppl 1):S61–5.

Gielen S, Adams V, Mobius-Winkles S, et al. Anti-inflammatory effects of exercise training in the skeletal muscle of patients with chronic heart failure. *J Am Coll Cardiol.* 2003 (Sept. 3);42(5):861–8.

Giovambattista A, Piermaria J, Suescun MO, et al. Direct effect of ghrelin on leptin production by cultured rat white adipocytes. *Obes Res.* 2006 (Jan);14(1):19–27.

Gnuidy SM. Obesity, metabolic syndrome, and coronary atherosclerosis. *Circulation*. 2002;23:2696–98.

Goode E. To curb cravings and even more. *New York Times*. April 15, 2003: F5.

Hill JO, Billington CJ. It's time to start treating obesity. *Am J Cardiol.* 2002 (April);89:969–72.

Hsueh, WA. A symposium: new insight into understanding the relation of type 2 diabetes mellitus, insulin resistance, and cardiovascular disease. *Supplement to the American Journal of Cardiology*: August 18, 2003.

Ioannou GN, Weiss NS, Boyko EJ, et al. Is central obesity a risk factor for cirrhosis-related death or hospitalization? A population-based cohort study. *Gastroenterology*. 2003;125(4):1053–9.

Isojarvi JI, Laatikainen TJ, Pakarinen AJ, et al. Polycystic ovaries and hyperandrogenism in women taking valproate for epilepsy. *N Engl J Med*. 1993;19:1383–88.

Isomaa B, Almgren P, Tuomi T et al. Cardiovascular morbidity and mortality associated with the metabolic syndrome. *Diabetes Care.* 2001;24:683–9.

Jadhav ST, Ferrell WR, Petrie JR, et al. Microvascular function, metabolic syndrome, and novel risk factor status in women with cardiac Syndrome X. *Am J Cardiology*. 2006 (June 15);97(12):1727–31.

Kloner RA. Introduction: Erectile dysfunction and cardiovascular risk factors. *Am J Cardiol.* 2003 (Nov. 6);92(9A):1–2.

Kolodny L. Erectile dysfunction and vascular disease. *Postgrad Med.* 2003 (Oct);114(4):30–4,39–40.

Kraus T, Haack M, Schuld A, et al. Body weight, the tumor necrosis factor system, and leptin production during treatment with mirtazapine or venlafaxine. *Pharmacopsychiatry.* 2002;35:220–5.

Krogh-Masen R, Plomgaard P. Insulin stimulates interleukin-6 and tumor necrosis factor gene expression in human subcutaneous adipose tissue. *Am J Physiol Endocrinol Metab*. 2004;286:E234–8.

Kumpusalo EA, Takala JK. Do beta-blockers put on weight? *Hypertension.* 2001;38(1):E4–5.

Lakka HM, Laaksonen DE, Lakka TA, et al. The metabolic syndrome and cardiovascular disease mortality in middle-aged men. *JAMA*. 2002;288:2709–16.

Lee KW, Lip GH. Effects of lifestyle on hemostasis, fibrinolysis, and platelet reactivity. *Arch Intern Med*. 2003;153:2368–92.

Lloyd CE, Wing RR, Orchard TJ. Waist-to-hip ratio and psychosocial factors in adults with insulin-dependent diabetes mellitus: the Pittsburgh Epidemiology of Diabetes Complications study. *Metabolism*. 1996 (Feb);45(2):268–72.

Loewinger LE, Young WB. Headache preventives: effect on weight. *Neurology*. 2002;58(suppl 3):A286.

Ludwig DS. The glycemic index, physiological mechanisms relating to obesity, diabetes, and cardiovascular disease. *JAMA*, 2002 (May 8);287(18):2414–23. Review.

Luef G, Abraham I, Haslinger M, et al. Polycystic ovaries, obesity and insulin resistance in women with epilepsy. A comparative study of carbamazepine and valproic acid in 105 women. *J Neurol*. 2002;7:835–41.

Maes M, Smith R, Christophe A, et al. Lower serum high-density lipoprotein cholesterol (HDL-C) in major depression and in depressed men with serious suicidal attempts: relationship with immune-inflammatory markers. *Acta Psyckiatr Scand*. 1997;95:212–21.

Masaki T, Yoshimatsu H, Chiba S, et al. Targeted disruption of histamine H-1 receptor attenuates regulatory effects of leptin on feeding, adiposity, and UCP family in mice. *Diabetes*. 2001;50(2):385–91.

Mechanisms for Metabolic Dysregulation Associated with Obesity. *Obesity*. 2006 (Feb);14(Suppl 1).

Meigs JB, D'Agostino RB Sr, Wilson PW, et al. Risk variable clustering in the insulin resistance syndrome. The Framingham Offspring study. *Diabetes*. 1997;46:1594–1600.

Meigs JB, Hu FB. Endothelial dysfunction predicts development of diabetes; *JAMA*. 2004; 291(16): 1978–86

Meigs JB. Epidemiology of the insulin resistance syndrome. *Curr Diabetes Rep*. 2003;3:73–9.

Miyatake N, Nishikawa H, Morishita A, et al. Daily walking reduces visceral adipose tissue areas and improves insulin resistance in Japanese obese subjects. *Diabetes Res Clin Pract.* 2002;58:101–7.

Mokdad AH, Ford ES, Bowman BA, et al. Prevalence of obesity, diabetes, and obesity-related health risk factors, 2001. *JAMA.* 2003;1:76–9.

Morley JE, Charlton E, Patrick P, et al. Validation of a screening questionnaire for androgen deficiency in aging males. *Metabolism.* 2000;49(9):1239–42.

Morris PJ, Packianatham, CI, Van Blerk CJ, Finer N. Moderate exercise and fibrinolytic potential in obese sedentary men with metabolic syndrome. *Obes Res.* 2003 (Nov);11(11):1333–8.

National Institutes of Health; National Heart, Lung, and Blood Institute; NHLBI Obesity Education Initiative; and the North American Association for the Study of Obesity. *The Practical Guide. Identification, evaluation, and treatment of overweight and obesity in adults.* October 2000;NIH Publication Number 00–4084. Available at: http://www.nhlbi.nih.gov/guidelines/obesity/practgde.htm.

Nemeroff CB. *Neuroendocrinology.* Boca Raton, FL: CRC Press; 1992; 618 pages.

Noppa H, Hallstrom T. Weight gain in adulthood in relation to socioeconomic factors, mental illness, and personality traits: a prospective study of middle-aged women. *J Psychosom Res.* 1981;25:83–9.

North American Association for the Study of Obesity, Supplement; Behavior Modification and Societal Change in the Prevention of Obesity; 2003 (Oct);11(Suppl).

O'Keefe JH, Cordain, L. Cardiovascular disease resulting from a diet and lifestyle at odds with our paleolithic genome: how to become a 21st century hunter-gatherer. *Mayo Clinic Proceedings.* 2004;79:101–8.

Pasini E, Aquilani R. Amino acids: chemistry and metabolism in normal and hypercatabolic states. *Am J Cardiol, Excerpta Medica:* April 2004.

Pavlou KN, Krey S, Steffee WP. Exercise as an adjunct to weight loss and maintenance in moderately obese subjects. *Am J Clin Nutr.* 1989;49:1115–23.

Pepine CJ. Integration of vascular biology. *Am J Cardiol, Excerpta Medica*: June 19, 2003.

Popkin BM, Neilsen SJ. The sweetening of the world's diet. *Obes Res*. 2003;11(11);1325–32.

Raggi PA. Symposium: Society of Atherosclerosis Imaging — Second International Meeting; *Supplement to the American Journal of Cardiology*. November 21, 2002.

Raikkonen K, Matthews KA, Kuller LH. The relationship between psychological risk attributes and the metabolic syndrome in healthy women: antecedent or consequence? *Metabolism*. 2002;51:1573–77.

Rasmussen MS, Lihn AS, Pedersen SB, et al. Adiponectin receptors in human adipose tissue: effects of obesity, weight loss, and fat depots. *Obesity*. 2006(Jan);14(1):28–35.

Rich-Edwards JW, Goldman MB, Willett WC, et al. Adolescent body mass index and infertility caused by ovulatory disorder. *Am J Obstet Gynecol*. 1994;171(1):171–2.

Roberts RE, Deleger S, Strawbridge WJ, Kaplan GA. Prospective association between obesity and depression: evidence from the Alameda County study. *Int J Obes Relat Metab Disord*. 2003;27:514–521.

Rosmond R, Bjorntorp P. Endocrine and metabolic aberrations in men with abdominal obesity in relation to arixio-depressive infirmity. *Metabolism*. 1998;47:1187–93.

Sajadieh A, Neilsen OW, Rasmussen V, et al. Increased heart rate and reduced heart-rate variability are associated with subclinical inflammation in middle-aged and elderly subjects with no apparaent heart disease. *Eur Heart J*. 2004 (Mar);25(5):363–70.

Sanyal AJ, Campbell, Sargent C, et al. Nonalcoholic steatohepatitis: association of insulin resistance and mitochondrial abnormalities. *Gastroenterology*. 2001;120:1183–92.

Selwyn AP, Popma JJ. Statins and the vascular wall: clinical and mechanistic correlates of early benefit. *Am J Cardiol, Excerpta Medica*: February 20, 2003.

Silja JV, Krsek M, et al. Angiogenic factors are elevated in overweight and obese individuals. *Int J Obes*. 2005;29:1308–14.

Sjostrom CD, Peltonen M, Wedel H, et al. Differentiated long-term effects of intentional weight loss on diabetes and hypertension. *Hypertension*. 2000; 36(1): 20–5.

Spector IE, Carey MP, Steinberg L. The sexual desire inventory: development, factor structure, and evidence of reliability. *Journal of Sex and Marital Therapy.* 1996; 22:175–90.

Stahl SM. Psychopharmacology Academy Syllabus, Vol. 1 & 2; 2003.

Sturmer T, Gunther KP, Brenner H. Obesity, overweight and patterns of osteoarthritis: the Ulm Osteoarthritis study. *J Clin Epidemiol.* 2000;53(3):307–13.

Talbot F, Nouwen A. A review of the relationship between depression and diabetes in adults: is there a link? *Diabetes Care.* 2000;23:1556–62.

Tracey KJ. The inflammatory reflex. *Nature.* 2002;420:853–9.

Wexler DJ, Hu FB, Manson GE, et al. Mediating effects of inflammatory biomarkers on insulin resistance associated with obesity. *Obes Res.* 2005 (Oct);13(10):1772–81.

Wolf AM, Colditz GA. Current estimates of the economic cost of obesity in the United States. *Obes Res* .1998;6:97–106.

Yamauchi MD, Moss KA, et al. Regulation of adiponectin expression in human adipocytes: effects of adiposity, glucocorticoids, and tumor necrosis factor. *Obesity.* 2005 (April);13(4):662–9.

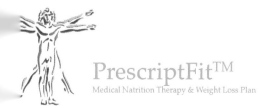

PrescriptFit™

Medical Natrition Therapy & Weight Loss Plan

PrescriptFit™ MNT Side Effects and Problem Solving

We know there are a number of obstacles you will face when making significant changes in eating habits and dietary changes. Some will involve changes to your environment, cooking more, avoiding familiar "fast" food solutions. Others will require a concentrated effort on the part of our whole family to support the changes you've decided to make. Each obstacle you face is important to understand and overcome to achieve improved health and quality life.

The section entitled, "Overcoming Obstacles" (pages 48 through 56), deals with many of the situational/psychological obstacles you may face as you begin the Amino Solution.

The tables on the following pages present at-a-glance information for dealing with the most common physical side effects our clinic patients have experienced related to making dietary changes and using the PrescriptFit™ amino acid supplements as shakes, soups, and puddings.

If these recommended solutions don't seem to resolve the problem you're experiencing, talk to your doctor about other medical conditions or treatments that could be the cause.

PHYSICAL PROBLEMS

	PROBABLE CAUSE	RECOMMENDED SOLUTION(S)
Intestinal Gas	A deficiency in an enzyme in the intestinal wall that normally breaks down complex carbohydrates (e.g., lactose containing PrescriptFit™ products) into simple sugars for digestion, causing intestinal bacteria to produce methane, butane, and formate gases	For 3 days, replace lactose containing PrescriptFit™ with seafood and poultry in Phases 2 & 3. Then start taking the lactose free PrescriptFit™ product. Gas should resolve within a day.
	Special Concerns/Related Info: Intestinal Gas — Those afflicted with Irritable Bowel Syndrome should only use only lactose-free PrescriptFit™ products. If you suffer from gas, read the disease section on Irritable Bowel Syndrome on pages 185 through 187.	
Diarrhea	Inadequate breakdown of complex carbohydrates in the intestine due to deficiency of enzymes. These undigested carbohydrates can: • Act just like a pile of sugar on the countertop will "suck" up an adjacent puddle of water: the high concentration of carbohydrate "sugar" in the intestine "sucks" water into the intestine, causing diarrhea. • Be converted by intestinal bacteria to toxic products (propionic acid) that irritate the intestinal lining, causing water and fluid to "leak" into the intestine to be expressed as diarrhea.	For 3 days, replace lactose containing PrescriptFit™ with seafood and poultry in Phases 2 & 3. Then start taking the **lactose free** PrescriptFit™ product. Diarrhea should not return.
	Special Concerns/Relation Information: Diarrhea — If diarrhea resolves after switching to lactose-free PrescriptFit™, it is likely that milk, fruit (and fruit juices), beans (legumes), and wheat products will also contribute to gas and diarrhea.	

	PROBABLE CAUSE	RECOMMENDED SOLUTION(S)
Constipation	A common problem due to decreased intake of fiber until Phase 4 (vegetables).	• Consume at least 8 glasses of water daily (e.g., unsweetened tea/soft drinks, water with shakes, etc) • Add fiber; the best sources are Citrucil (tablets or powder), Metamucil, or other OTC fiber products. • Use a laxative, preferably a stool softner (e.g, Surfak OTC or Milk of Magnesia). • Take a fish oil supplement (up to 6 tablets/day).
	Special Concerns/Relation Information: Constipation — *Daily laxatives should not be necessary.*	
Nausea	Nausea can occur either as: • A common symptom of gallstones or stomach ulcers. • An aversion response — something avoided because of an unpleasant experience. In the latter case, nausea typically begins only with the start of the "diet," whereas symptoms will exist prior to the "diet" with the former scenario.	Nausea should be addressed medically. Tests for gallstones or stomach ulcers should be considered. If negative, your physician can prescribe Reglan 10 mg prior to each amino acid shake for 1–2 weeks. Results will be immediate if Reglan works. Another option is to discontinue PrescriptFit™ shakes for 2 weeks while continuing foods in Phases 2 or higher to see if symptoms continue.
	***Special Concerns/Relation Information: Nausea** — Nausea is most common in carbohydrate-addicted individuals (see page 13–15 for more information on carbohydrate addiction). **Ask your doctor** about taking Wellbutrin XL and then re-trying PrescriptFit™. Wellbutrin is FDA approved for use as an antidepressant or anti-anxiety agent as well as for cigarette addiction. Food addiction has many of the same brain characteristics as cigarette addiction.*	

	Probable Cause	Recommended Solution(s)
Weakness/Lightheadedness	Fluid loss that causes a drop in blood pressure. Excess fluid weight loss of 8-10 pounds is very common after the first week of the PrescriptFit™ MNT Plan. **Talk to your doctor BEFORE beginning the PrescriptFit™ MNT Plan if currently taking medication to reduce fluid (diuretics) or lower blood pressure (antihypertensives).**	• Consume all recommended PrescriptFit™ doses mixed as shakes with adequate volumes of water. Drink 4-8 additional glasses/servings of water or non-caloric soft drinks, tea, or flavored water daily. • **With physician supervision ONLY**, discontinue or reduce medication intake for fluid retention and high blood pressure. • Use PrescriptFit™ Chicken or Beef Soups that contain some salt to retain water and raise blood pressure. • Advance to Phase 2 or 3 (seafood or poultry), and season with salt to retain water and raise blood pressure.

Special Concerns/Relation Information: Weakness/Lightheadedness — Those taking diuretic, high blood pressure, or any other medication that lowers blood pressure need contact their doctor immediately if weakness or lightheadedness occur. For more information, review the sections on hypertension (pages 176 through 179) and hyperlipidemia (pages 172 through 175).

Hypoglycemia/Feeling "Shaky"	Taking medications that lower blood sugar (for type 2 diabetes). Talk to your doctor BEFORE beginning the PrescriptFit™ MNT Plan if currently taking any medication to reduce blood sugar.	• With physician supervision ONLY, reduce prescribed medications, such as insulin or glyburide. • Quickly consume additional PrescriptFit™ supplements or snack bars to reduce symptoms within 5-15 minutes. • Consume 8 or more doses of PrescriptFit™ products daily.

Special Concerns/Relation Information: Hypoglycemia/Feeling "Shaky" — Those treated for diabetes must monitor their blood sugar at least once a day in Phases 1 and 2 of the Plan and keep in close contact with their doctor. Occasionally, weakness from low blood pressure (as described above) is mistaken for hypoglycemia. When in question, consume more PrescriptFit™ and more fluids. For more information on diabetes, review pages 165 through 167.

	PROBABLE CAUSE	RECOMMENDED SOLUTION(S)
Tiredness/Loss of Energy	Inadequate dosing of the PrescriptFit™ amino acid products to save money or calories. Problems with sleep patterns, exercise extremes, and other medical causes, including side effects of medication.	• Consume more PrescriptFit™ doses daily by combining 2–4 doses in each serving. • Talk to your doctor about other possible causes for your loss of energy unrelated to your diet.

Special Concerns/Relation Information: Tiredness/Loss of Energy — If tiredness fails to resolve by adding more PrescriptFit™ doses per day, it is probably not from lack of food.

	PROBABLE CAUSE	RECOMMENDED SOLUTION(S)
Hunger/Cravings	Some confuse hunger with cravings. Cravings or "compulsion" is a feeling of "hunger" unrelated to the need for food. This form of food addiction or dependency occurs frequently during Phase 1 or 2 of the PrescriptFit™ MNT Plan.	Quickly consume 2–4 doses of PrescriptFit™ amino acids in a single or multiple shakes, puddings, or soups. If the "hunger" does not resolve, it is most likely a craving or food addiction issue. "Retrain" your brain by feeding yourself more doses of PrescriptFit™ every time a craving or feeling of hunger occurs. Your brain will quickly learn that every "craving" feeling is followed by another shake, pudding, or soup rather than the usual chocolate, pastry, or pasta. Soon your "hungry" brain will learn adapt and stop harassing you with cravings. Move immediately to the next Phase, which will "trick" your brain into accepting a "reward" that is less than expected. Keep advancing to other Phases until the cravings subside. Then go back to an earlier Phase associated with more rapid weight loss and disease control, advancing forward again to the next Phases on schedule. Ask your doctor about medications used to treat addictive behavior.

Special Concerns/Relation Information: Hunger/Cravings — Oddly enough, hunger — true hunger — is rarely experienced on the PrescriptFit™ MNT Plan. With proper doses, you get adequate protein and carbohydrate in the additional branched chain amino acids to avoid behavior changes, including hunger. Those who first admit they have an addiction to food can begin to treat and overcome that addiction. For more information, review the material on sugar addiction on pages 13 through 15.

The Amino Solution
©2009 Stanford A. Owen, MD

	Probable Cause	Recommended Solution(s)
Muscle Fatigue/Cramps	**Muscle Fatigue:** Low carbohydrate diets coupled with exhaustive exercise can cause sugar depletion in the muscles after 30–40 minutes of such exercise. Also known as "runner's fatigue."	• Consume PrescriptFit™ supplements within 60 minutes of completing exhaustive exercise. • Increase dosage of PrescriptFit™ shakes, soup, or puddings.
	Muscle Cramps: Either depletion of muscle-storage sugar or potassium (typically from taking diuretics during initial phase of the Plan when fluid loss is most likely). Low potassium levels cause heart rhythm irritability and even heart muscle failure (a heart "cramp"). PrescriptFit™ MNT uses complex carbohydrates found in non-fat milk solids to prevent muscle cramps.	• **See you doctor and monitor potassium levels carefully** if taking diuretic medication (even if recently discontinued). • Take a potassium supplement as prescribed by your doctor.

Special Concerns/Relation Information: Muscle Fatigue/Cramps — *Muscles contain only a limited amount of readily available stored sugar, known as glycogen. After depletion, a small time "window" of rapid repletion of muscle sugar occurs from dietary consumption, lasting 15–60 minutes after the exhaustive exercise. If sugar is not consumed and presented to the glycogen-depleted muscle during that "window," the muscle never quite recovers 100 percent. The next day, the muscle doesn't perform as well. If the sugar "window" is again missed, even more muscle depletion occurs resulting in tiredness and fatigue, requiring rest and recovery. Muscle sugar-depletion is aggravated further if you begin or increase exercise during the low-carb phase of a diet.*

The Amino Solution
©2009 Stanford A. Owen, MD

INDEX

PRODUCTS

Available online at www.drdiet.com or by calling 888-460-6286.

PrescriptFit™ Shakes, Soups, Puddings

Vanilla	Beef
Chocolate	Chicken
Lactose Free Vanilla	
Lactose Free Chocolate	

PrescriptFit™ Snack Bars

Double Chocolate	Chocolate Mint
Toffee	Oatmeal Cinnamon Raisin
Brownie Bar	Peanut Butter Crunch
Butter Pecan w/ Caramel	Peanut Butter
Lemon Crunch	Chocolate Chip Cookie Dough
CrispN'Crunch Cinnamon	Cookies and Cream
CrispN'Crunch Peanut	CrispN'Crunch Double Berry
CrispN'Crunch Fudge Graham	CrispN'Crunch Cocoa Cafe

Flavors

Butter Pecan	Strawberry
Mint Chocolate	Mocha
Orange Cream	Black Rasberry
Banana Coconut	Caramel
Cake Batter	Mango
Chocolate Fudge	

PrescriptFit™ Educational Material

The Amino Solution	The Weighing Game
PrescriptFit™ Calendar	The Best Sex Book

The Amino Solution
©2009 Stanford A. Owen, MD